W0228108

MODERN GERIATRICS SERIES

Series Editor: J. Wedgwood

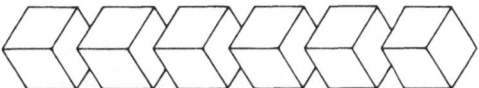

FITS, FAINTS AND FALLS IN OLD AGE

MODERN GERIATRICS SERIES

Series Editor: J. Wedgwood

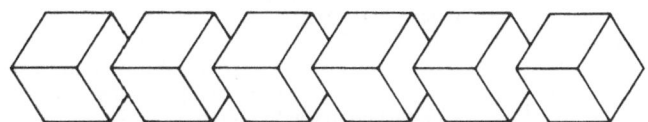

FITS, FAINTS AND FALLS IN OLD AGE

Edited by Mohan S. Kataria

Department of General Medicine for the Elderly
St. Mary's Hospital, Luton

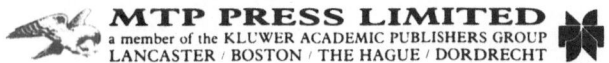

MTP PRESS LIMITED
a member of the KLUWER ACADEMIC PUBLISHERS GROUP
LANCASTER / BOSTON / THE HAGUE / DORDRECHT

Published in the UK and Europe by
MTP Press Limited
Falcon House
Lancaster, England

British Library Cataloguing in Publication Data
Fits, faints and falls in old age.—(Modern
 geriatrics series)
 1. Geriatric neurology
 I. Kataria, Mohan S.   II. Series
 618.97′68   RC346

Published in the USA by
MTP Press
A division of Kluwer Boston Inc
190 Old Derby Street
Hingham, MA 02043, USA

Library of Congress Cataloging in Publication Data
Main Entry under Title:
(Modern Geriatrics Series)
Includes Bibliographies and index.
1. Geriatrics.   2. Falls (Accidents)
3. Locomotion, Disordered.   4. Neurological Manifesta-
tions of General Diseases.   5. Brain – Diseases –
Complications and Sequelae.   I. Kataria, Mohan S.
II. Series.   [DNLM: 1. Gait – In Old Age.
2. Locomotion – In Old Age.   3. Neurologic Manifestations
– In Old Age.   4. Seizures – In Old Age.   5. Syncope –
In Old Age.   WL 340 F546]
RC952.5.F57 1985   617′.1′0080565   85-10318

ISBN-13: 978-94-010-8666-0   e-ISBN-13: 978-94-009-4892-1
DOI: 10.1007/978-94-009-4892-1

Copyright © 1985 MTP Press Limited
Softcover reprint of the hardcover 1st edition 1985
All rights reserved. No part of this publication
may be reproduced, stored in a retrieval
system, or transmitted in any form or by any
means, electronic, mechanical, photocopying,
recording or otherwise, without prior permission
from the publishers.

Contents

CONTENTS

List of Contributors

D. BAYLISS
Occupational Therapy Department
King's College Hospital
Denmark Hill
London SE5
ENGLAND

K. G. F. BENTON
Department of Medicine for the
    Elderly
St Helen's Hospital
Hastings
East Sussex
ENGLAND

S. K. DAS
Department of Geriatric Medicine
St Helier Group of Hospitals
St Helier Hospital
Wrythe Lane
Carshalton
Surrey SM5 1AA
ENGLAND

A. J. D. FARQUHARSON
Department of Geriatric Medicine
Orsett Hospital
Grays
Essex RM16 3EV
ENGLAND

M. GREEN
Department of Geriatric Medicine
New End Hospital
Hampstead
London NW3
ENGLAND

M. S. KATARIA
Department of General Medicine for
    the Elderly
South Bedfordshire Health Authority
St Mary's Hospital
Dunstable Road
Luton LU1 1BE
ENGLAND

P. W. OVERSTALL
Department of Age Care
General Hospital
Hereford HR1 2PA
ENGLAND

A. SQUIRES
Department of Physiotherapy
Dulwich Hospital North Wing
St Francis Road
Dulwich
London SE22 8DF
ENGLAND

T. M. STROUTHIDIS
Department of Medicine for the
    Elderly
St Helen's Hospital
Hastings
East Sussex
ENGLAND

Preface

Events in any one day of the aged consist of the functions of daily living modified or enhanced for each individual according to his or her capability. It is the constant aim of the medical professions to enhance the individual's quality of life and to try to avoid what is preventable.

Among some of the hazards of the geriatric day are fits, faints and falls.

It is the fall which often highlights the first two and the consequences may be serious for an old person. Perhaps one day an easy way to circumvent the 'forces of gravity' or drugs to counteract impaired sensory input will be found.

The importance of the study of gait has been increasingly recognized by physicians working in this field of medicine for the elderly; writings by geriatricians on the subject are numerous. Bernard Isaacs in his gait research laboratory in Birmingham is studying the subject.

In this book the experience of the contributors is brought together, inevitably with some overlap, which has in the main been avoided by restructuring, modification and crosschecking of articles.

Initially we sat down together at the Dulwich Golf Club to draw up a list of subjects and headings under which fits, falls and faints were to be broadly treated. However, the hazards of collating the various contributions can be legion. One contributor had his manuscript and money stolen while abroad; another found himself in the middle of a move to a different appointment, while yet another found himself elevated to the status of a 'senior citizen' and all that goes with the transition. In spite of all this the book somehow materialized.

We did not set out to write just another textbook on this subject, but we hope that this book will complement the present excellent accounts in some general medicine textbooks.

Many of the situations discussed in this book may be equally applicable to the younger person but with less resultant falls and less serious consequences.

Medicine is now treated as a 'holistic discipline'. To add another dimension to it would be to recognize that philosophy and science are having to come together as nature yields the secrets of the cosmos and the atom. Things may appear different to the observer depending on where he or she stands.

I am indebted to my colleagues who have collaborated and helped in this venture. It has been a privilege and a pleasure to work with them. One always learns from one's patients, colleagues and students, and I take this opportunity to thank them.

Finally, I wish to thank our Series Editor, Dr John Wedgwood, for valuable advice; and Martin Lister of MTP Press whom I found always friendly and willing to help.

Mohan S. Kataria
Kings College Hospital
and
St Francis Hospital, 1985

Series Editor's Note

This series attempts to keep abreast of developments in Geriatric Medicine. This is no easy task in such a rapidly expanding subject.

The editors of each volume and their authors have approached the subject from the point of view of practising clinicians, experienced in what can now be called the British tradition of Geriatric Medicine. The text is aimed at those wishing to acquire a more specialised knowledge of Geriatric Medicine either in hospital or in general practice. At the same time it is hoped that it will be of value to both undergraduate and postgraduate students.

Nevertheless, it has been said that we 'all practise geriatrics now', and, bearing in mind the kernel of truth in this observation, it is hoped that this series will be of interest to an even wider medical readership.

The Series Editor has always favoured a multi-disciplinary approach to training in Geriatric Medicine, and hopes that this slant will also allow the Series to be of value to our colleagues in the para-medical and nursing professions.

The first volume deals with acute geriatric medicine, a subject which has become of particular importance with the emergency admission policies of a number of geriatric units today, and the combination of general and general medical 'firms'.

The second volume deals with the difficult problem of fits, faints and falls in the old.

The next to follow will be about infections in the elderly.

John Wedgewood, MA, MD, FRCP

1

The Human Walk and Fall

M. S. KATARIA

INTRODUCTION

Mobility is one of the essential requirements of modern life, and falls and immobility are probably the most common reasons for medical intervention in the elderly.

To fully understand human locomotion and the consequences of its derangement, the normal mechanism as well as the development of the bipedal status must be considered. Human mobility is undoubtedly one of the most important functions upon which natural selection has operated.

Locomotion is a characteristic of animal life. Progression is a sequence of processes by which the animal moves, from one location to another, and is determined by many interrelated factors. The basic incentives may be food, fight and flight; a few animals use their olfactory apparatus to follow pheromones to find a mate. Animals need organic nutrition, so they require a mechanism for mobility and well-developed sensors to seek out their food. However, human beings move for considerably more reasons.

BASIC REQUIREMENTS FOR SAFE WALKING

The following are necessary to initiate the action of walking.

1. Will and orientation.
2. Supportive structure.
3. Continuous support against gravity.
4. Proper proprioceptive and postural control.
5. Alternating rhythmic motion of head, limbs and trunk.

A SHORT HISTORY OF EVOLUTION

The evolution of mammals was punctuated by a series of fundamental adaptations as they adjusted to changes in environment and lifestyle. One particularly significant phase of vertebrate evolution may be summarized as follows.

The Crossopterygian

The crossopterygian – a 1.5 metre fish with a lobed front fin – crawled out of the salt water on to swampy land, and using its fins groped its way from one brackish waterhole to the next. This radical change from seawater to land atmosphere required a large number of physical adaptations in order to keep the biochemistry and the internal milieu of the creature's body in equilibrium. Animals which survived the change of environment were those which succeeded in keeping their calcium, phosphate, sodium and potassium in balance. They also had to perfect the art of breathing through nostrils into the air bladders (lungs) which supplied their bodies with oxygen.

Towards Homo sapiens

According to Darwin and his successors, the evolution of primates towards *Homo sapiens* was a multistage process that took millions of years. Among the basic forces that determined our physical evolution was the change from a quadrupedal to a bipedal stance which needed strong bones and responsive muscles.

About ten million years ago, in the Rift valley of western Kenya, the pro-hominid stage occurred. The habitual carrying of food and other burdens had forced these missing links into bipedal progression. Feet became flatter; the big toes were rotated and began to lie parallel with the other toes, providing stability for upright stance, and ankles consequently became strengthened. The knees rotated inwards to lie below the midline of the hips. The pelvis became narrowed and strengthened to bear the weight of the body. Unlike their ancestors these creatures no longer swayed from side to side as they walked. *Homo sapiens*, by standing on two hind-legs, released the two front limbs for a prehensile role in performing hunter–killer–gatherer tasks. The opposition of the thumb gave a dramatically improved hand performance in accomplishing intricate work. Together with these changes the frontal lobes have progressively developed as an area subserving intellectual control and speech. These changes have helped to conquer nature. The use of tools, in addition, may at the same time be both cause and effect of bipedal locomotion.

The human line of vision lies along the longitudinal axis of the head which is at right angles to the neck. Thus the bipedal stance is necessary for effective vision. A dog's line of vision lies along the longitudinal direction of its head, in the same line as its neck and spine, and is thus compatible with its quadruped status (Figure 1.1). Facial shortening, therefore, was a vital development in the progression to bipedalism. Changes in the last 300

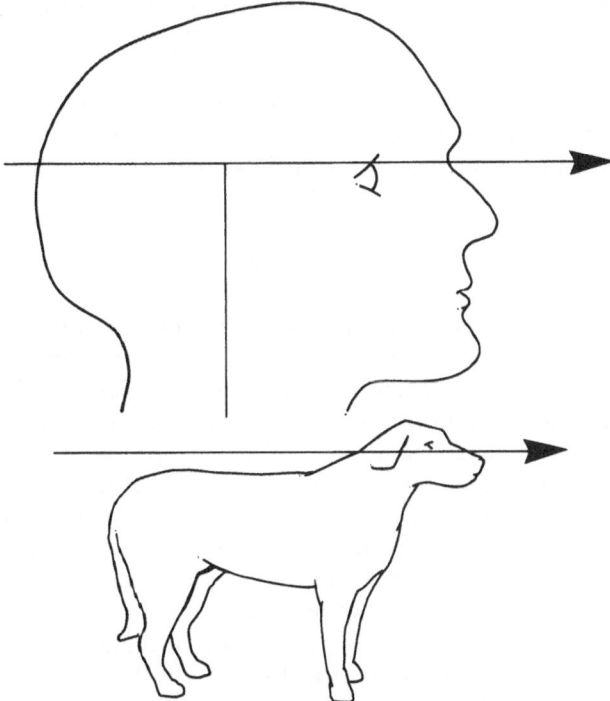

Figure 1.1 Line of vision in relation to the axis of the spine in the human and the dog

million years have been those of proportion rather than in the addition of new elements. The increase in size of the frontal lobes has been one of the most significant changes.

The reptilian advance is effected in many cases by a lateral flexion and extension of its spine. The 'galant' reflex of the infant – whereby it flexes its body to the side which is gently stroked – is a postural reflex which later disappears. The bipedal stance, however, relieved the spine of its locomotor duty; the bony spine had to remain pliable so it became jointed. The majority of mammals are quadripeds and have three legs on the ground at any time during slow walking; the human infant more or less does the same thing while crawling. However, when standing on two legs the infant's proprioceptive reflex systems must adjust to walking on two legs.

CENTRE OF GRAVITY AND BALANCE

In the resting state, balance is the state of equilibrium of the body with its environment. During action, balance is still achieved by the maintenance of this equilibrium. Most four-footed animals can stand on their hind-legs, but then the segments of these hind-legs have to remain partially flexed in relation to one another.

As long as the centre of gravity falls within the base formed by the two feet the erect body remains in equilibrium. The spinal changes in modern man have allowed the centre of gravity of the trunk to be brought back to a line above the acetabula, resulting in a lumbar lordosis peculiar solely to humans. The extensor muscles of the knee, hip and trunk play an important part in producing man's upright position.

STRIDE AND GAIT

The human stride was accompanied by a shorter hip bone and an increase in the size of the femoral head. There was also a concomitant increase in cranial capacity and consequently in the size of the female birth canal. This in time increased the femoral angle and shortened the femoral neck. The striding gait, the ability to stand erect with straight lower limbs, or to stand for long periods in balance without expenditure of much energy, and the ability to walk long distances, are some especially human characteristics.

Individuals acquire their own individual style of locomotion and gait pattern which distinguishes them even from a distance. People are often recognized by the particular sound of their footsteps, rather like a signature tune. There is a basic pattern of progression, consisting of a continuous 'make and break' of the line of the body's centre of gravity during forward propulsion.

The line of advance is governed by the will, direction of the eyes and head, hip flexion, and inclination of the body in the intended direction. A plumb line from the body of the second sacral vertebra usually lies along the line of the centre of gravity. The hip joint is slightly anterior to this line and knee and ankle joints slightly behind. The stable stance – both feet on the ground – is the neutral state.

The movement forward – for example, of the right leg after 'toe off' – upsets the balance and while the body rests on the left leg a succession of associated adjustments take place. The length of the stride is increased by medial rotation and tilt of the hip towards the side of the supporting limb. As the upper left arm swings forward, the upper spine rotates towards the right, thus equalizing the hip rotation. In the female, due to anatomical differences, there is exaggeration of all the associated movements while achieving the stride, thus adding allure to the advance. As the right heel strikes the ground there is a return to the transient state of both feet touching the ground. During one cycle of one lower limb – for instance, toe off to heel strike – both feet touch the ground together twice, and the body and limbs are in state of dynamic equilibrium. This human progression provides a striking contrast to the advance of the 'robot', where the spine and pelvis are rigid and only the legs and arms advance alternately and stiffly.

Disability due to disease or defect disturbs normal gait. Thus the study of gait may provide much information, particularly in the diagnosis of neurological disease.

WHY WE FALL

No animal exists or can survive independent of its own environment. The animal which utilizes environmental resources must also be able to adjust to it and cope with its inherent hazards.

During the process of evolution many may have inherited and stored in their subconscious some of the fears and complexes acquired on the way. For example, the infant baboon appears to be born with three fears – falling, snakes, and the dark. Of these the fear of falling is still paramount in humans especially in the elderly.

As a result of psychological, cardiorespiratory, musculoskeletal and psychiatric disorders motor function can be affected. This becomes apparent in the altered attitude of the affected person. The stable stance of an individual is the sum total of active postural and proprioceptive, vagal and labyrinthine reflexes that lock and maintain the skeleton in an erect posture. Alteration of the centre of gravity sets in motion various reflexes to harmonize and counterbalance the result of this disturbance by the advancing step. The assurance of a safe stance and stride is the very basis of the prevention of falls, and hence often survival.

The pressure of the feet on the ground and proprioceptive reflexes generated thereby are some of the most important factors in stability. Progression, therefore, is like music from a sensitive and responsive orchestra, harmonizing the various components that form part of it. Normally a good conductor is capable of adjusting to malfunction of parts when this capacity is impaired or lost, and the music becomes discordant. Similarly balance can be disturbed by disease or disability of the nervous, optical, auditory, and musculoskeletal systems.

Normally, walking is more or less an automatic act, so when it becomes conscious accidents are likely to happen, as is suggested by the following

> The centipede was happy quite until the frog for fun
> Said 'Pray which leg goes after which?'
> Which wrought him up to such a pitch
> He lay distracted in a ditch
> Considering how to run.

To restore this automacity is one of the goals of rehabilitation.

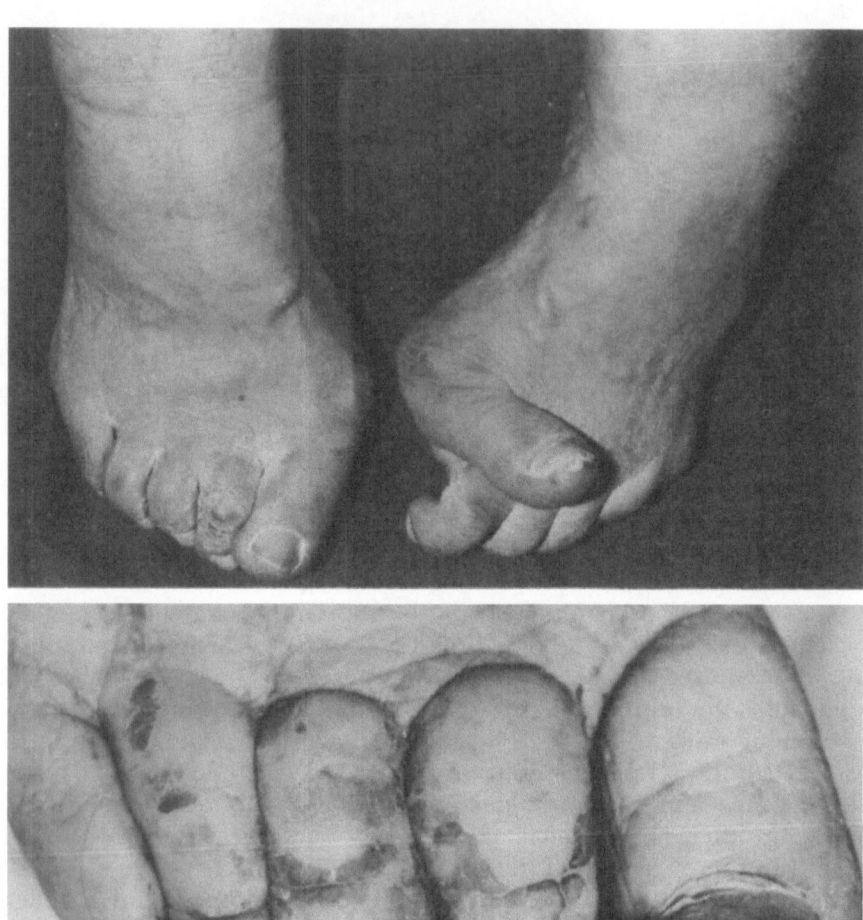

Figure 1.2 (a) and (b) Some mechanical and destabilizing factors. (a) hallux valgus; (b) onychogryphosis; (c) severe kyphosis osteoporosis; (d) genu recurvatum; (e) Paget's disease of the tibia; (f) genu valgum; (g) osteoma of the femur; (h) lymphoedema – 'heavy legs'.

ANATOMY OF FALLS

An accident is an unforeseen event. A fall may be due to the failure of the normal antigravity and compensatory mechanisms of the supportive dynamic architecture, proprioception and changes in force of the effect of the

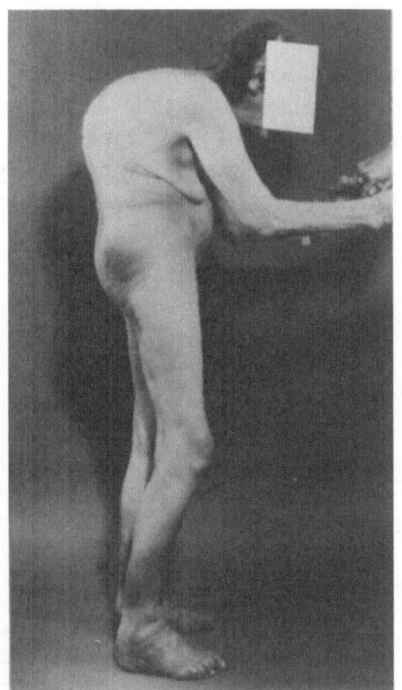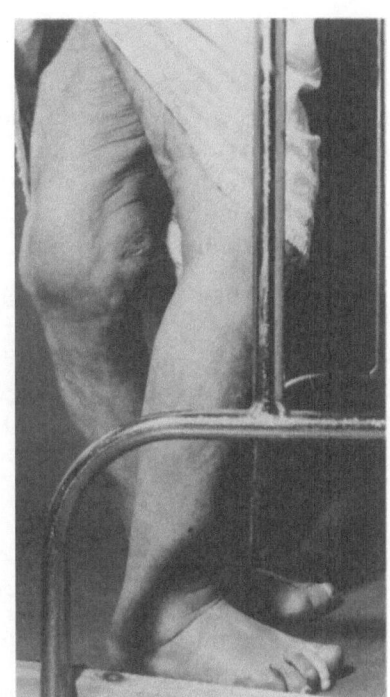

Figure 1.2 (c) and (d)

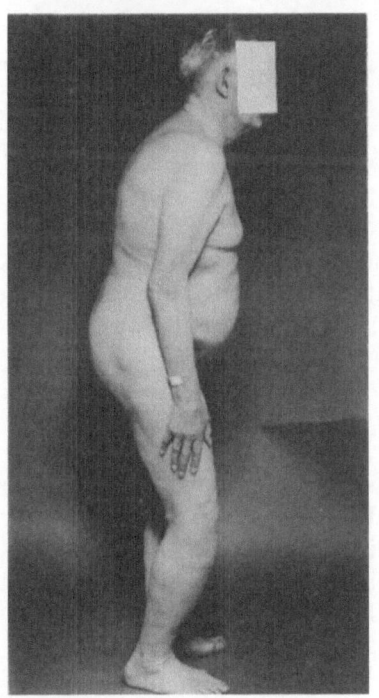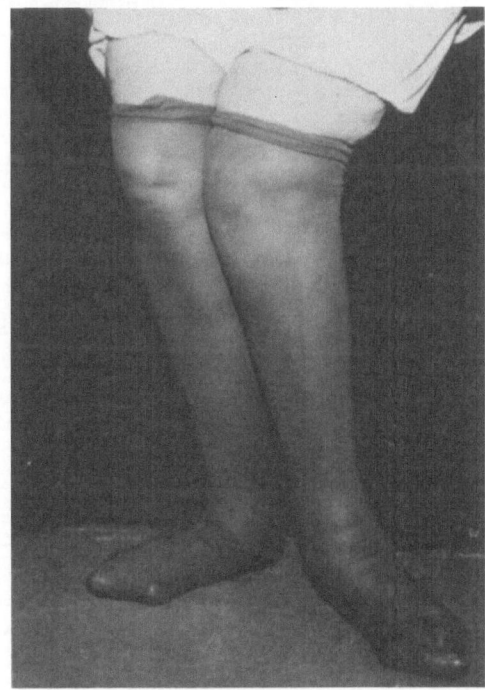

Figure 1.2 (e) and (f)

centre of gravity on an individual. Physical deformity of the architecture of the body may be conducive to the loss of balance and falls. Psychological factors and inattention may, however, also play an important role.

The body architecture in its normal dynamic state is supported by the normal functioning and control of biochemical, vascular, neurological, metabolic, and physical factors.

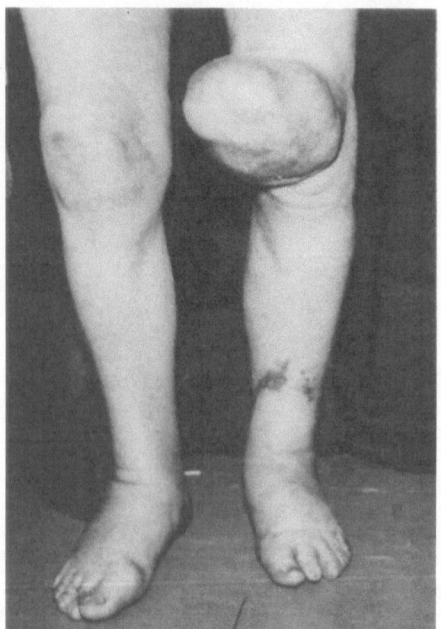 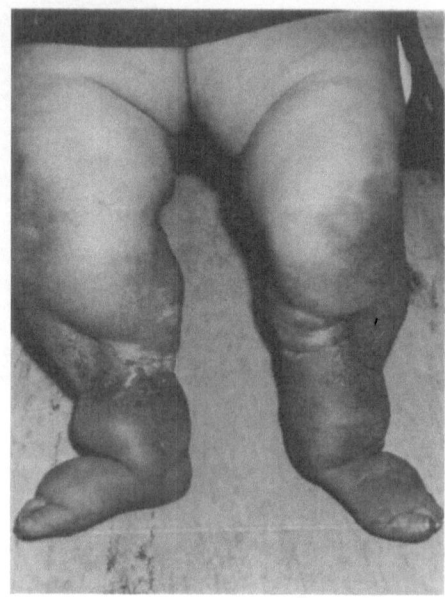

Figure 1.2 (g) and (h)

The cause of dysfunction may be in the head, neck, heart, or limbs. There is a risk of falling during altered state of control of proprioception, due to, for example, a confused or twilight state (that is, half awake) due to drugs, intoxicants, or poisons – internal or external.

How We Fall

Kinetic (internal or external) fall ⟨ Push
Pull
Spiral, for example, vertigo
Failed rectification (stagger reflex), after trip or fall
Festinant, forward, back or lateral, for example, Parkinson's disease

The following may cause falls:

1. The body may lose balance while running and fall.
2. There could be a kinetic collapse – folding at the knees, hips and body, such as in a faint.
3. A rigid body fall (or falling like a log) could be caused by Parkinsonism, lost postural control, or tonic state of grand mal epilepsy.

After We Fall

The patient's history should be taken and a thorough examination made. First any immediate condition that needs attention is dealt with. In case of fractures there should be a joint approach to management between physician and orthopaedic surgeon. When the patient is ready, observation and analysis of gait, the condition of the feet, nails and footwear are necessary for diagnosis and to plan treatment. A team programme can then be worked out with the participation of the patient.

After a fall the elderly are often unable to get off the floor, due to, for example, obesity, weakness, arthritis, stroke or loss of righting reflexes. This group of the elderly particularly runs the risk of hypothermia or dehydration after prolonged exposure to cold.

There are many alarm devices which can be carried on the person, to enable the victim to summon help. Recently a 'rescue chair'* has been devised and made, where if the person can drag herself or himself on to the seat, a push button on the chair raises the seat, bringing the person to a sitting position. From here, by pressing the feet firmly on the ground, it is possible to stand up.

ASSESSMENT

Treatment, management, discharge and placement with follow-up requires the by now well-recognized joint expertise of the multidisciplinary team and the skill of the geriatrician. An aide-memoire which may be helpful is given below:

C is the patient *continent*?
A is the patient *ambulant*?
R is the patient *rational*?
D is the patient able to *dress himself/herself*?
S is the patient motivated and has he/she *somewhere to go*?

Persistence and morale are two important factors in the rehabilitation of the patient. When a certain poet politician was asked how his country had

* Rehabilitation Products, Bridge Works, Hasketon, Woodridge, Suffolk.

managed to achieve independent status (applicable to patients struggling to be independent) he said:

'Simply this is how –
We woke up, we sat up and we got up,
We walked a baby step or two and fell.
We got up and walked again,
Falling and walking; cheered and praised,
This is how we got walking' (Translation – Author)

Bibliography

Bronowski, J. (1973). *The Ascent of Man.* (London: BBC Publications)

Cosgrove, M. (1969). *Bone for Bone.* (London: Lutterworth Press)

Das, S. K. and Kataria, M. S. (1984). Prevention of accidents in the home. *Age Int.*, **2** (1)

Evans, D. P. (1982). *Backache: its Evolution and Conservative Treatment.* (Lancaster: MTP Press)

Kataria, M. S. and Squires, A. (1983). A step by step guide to defying gravity. *Ther. Week.*, **February 17**

Purdon Martin, J. (1967). *The Basal Ganglia and Posture.* (London: Pitman Medical)

Roaf, R. (1977). *Posture.* (London: Academic Press)

Sagan, C. (1978). *The Dragons of Eden.* (London: Hodder and Stoughton)

2

Stability, Movement and Posture

S. K. DAS and M. S. KATARIA

STABILITY AND MOVEMENT

Adjustment from the quadruped status to the bipedal mode of locomotion has added the hazard of falling to all the other consequences of the change, which may be anything from flat feet, osteoarthritis, herniae, prolapsed discs and kyphosis, down to an ordinary trip fall.

The uncertain steps of a child beginning to walk are the learning processes whereby the cerebrum, cerebellum and postural reflexes are beginning to coordinate for the practice of locomotion. At this stage walking is not yet the automatic, effortless, subconscious mechanism whereby adults move when learning is complete.

It takes about 18 months for the pyramidal system to develop to the stage when Babinski's reflex changes from positive (upgoing toe) to normal flexor response. The postural reflexes are mediated through the spinal and cerebellar tracts and are constantly informed through the eyes, ears (semicircular canals), muscles, joints and the skin. The relationship of the body to the surrounding objects and environment also exerts its regulatory influence.

So naturally the central and peripheral mechanisms of posture keep the body balanced and vertical unless we will it otherwise. Adult vertical *Homo sapiens* keeps on balance while walking along without having to think about it.

The body is in a dynamic situation and does not behave merely as a mass on two sticks. Extreme ageing and/or disease changes in the mechanisms put these protective reflexes at risk with consequent failure and falls. The young may be able to get off lightly with minor bruising. However, for the elderly the results of falls can be disastrous.

Biomechanics and Kinesiology of Human Body Movement

Movement of any object depends on the resultant forces acting on the body. The study of these movements in the living human body is called biomechanics, and it depends on both statics (that is, concerned with bodies in balance) and dynamics (that is, concerned with bodies in motion).

In biomechanics motion constitutes the force, and force mostly depends on movement. In the human body such force and movement is controlled by a process of equilibrium, that is, through sensory apparatus, posterior columns, cerebellum, vestibular apparatus and joint sense.

Apart from this, the balancing mechanism of the human body also depends on the weight of the individual, because in biomechanics weight is the force with which the human body is attracted towards the earth by the gravitational attraction, expressed in mathematics as $W = M \times G$ where W = weight, M = mass, and G = force of gravity (failure of equation equals fall).

POSTURE – PULL AND PROGRESSION

The erect human posture is often held to have been achieved at the cost of such a protracted evolution that it can be considered prone to all manner of drawbacks, and results in frequent breakdown and subsequent pathological changes in the weight-bearing joints.

The human primate is singular in his bipedal posture – mechanically unstable when compared with its height, and with a mechanically minimal support base. As such, a slight alteration or displacement of the trunk from its vertical position puts the human body into a state of disequilibrium.

In the normal static phase the centre of gravity of any segment of the body substantially falls above the joints upon which its weight rests. Even the head is almost, if not wholly, balanced upon the atlanto-occipital joint and cervical spinal column.

In most individuals (when standing erect) the vertical centre of gravity also stretches along the hips and knees till it ends in the earth. It thus tends to increase tension in the plantar arches in flexion and soleus-gastrocnemius muscles to prevent a forward sway or actual fall. Thus, such an erect posture in extension can be maintained for a certain period provided that the servomechanism of the body remains in balance. The sensor of servomechanism which maintains balance has visual, vestibular, and proprioceptive elements through long tracts of the central nervous system. The erect posture in extension is maintained by long tracts, especially the lateral column, but the maintenance of the servomechanism to keep the body in balance consists of posterior columns and its proprioceptive sensor, with their connection to the brain stem, cerebellum, basal ganglia and the motor cortex as the afferent connections. The efferent component (to maintain the balance) is usually carried out as an outflow tract from the motor and sensory cortex through the spinal cord and peripheral nerves to the muscles. In locomotion, especially in the swing phase, whether it be walking, running or jumping, the centre of gravity – vertical sensor – is displaced from its stable position but takes a coordinated posture; for example, the toes leave the ground as the opposite heel meets it to transfer support. The trailing leg, relieved of weight-bearing, swings forward with slight flexion at the hip and knee, dorsiflexion of the foot and a pendular action of the hip flexors. As the limit of the stride is reached, the momentum of the limb is overcome by the hip extensor to bring the heel to the ground, and therefore to begin another cycle.

Repeated falls in the elderly are part of a symptom complex which requires investigation. About 34% of all falls in the elderly are due to accidental interruption of the cycle of locomotion as described (Backett, 1965; Sheldon, 1960).

Analysis of all falls shows that there is only one reason why human beings fall forward, backward or sideways; this is basically due to alteration of the centre of gravity of the body, resulting in loss of balance.

Most injury will depend on the speed of force with which the fall occurred; it may not affect the total body but will be proportional to the movement of the body, relative to whether the movement is slow or rapid.

References

Backett, E. M. (1965). *Domestic Accidents*. (Geneva: World Health Organization)
Sheldon, J. H. (1960). On the natural history of falls in old age. *Br. Med. J.*, **2**, 1685–90

3

Epidemiology and Pathophysiology of Falls

P. W. OVERSTALL

PREVALENCE

Surveys of elderly persons living in their own homes show that about a
third give a history of a fall during the previous 12 months (Exton-Smith,
1977; Prudham and Evans, 1981; Sheldon, 1948). There is an increasing
prevalence of falls with age and a higher rate of falls among females than
males. In the 65–69 age-group the prevalence of falls is about 13% for
males and 30% for females, and rises in the 80–84 age-group to 33% and
44% respectively. In those aged 85 years and over a decreased prevalence
has been noted both in men (Exton-Smith, 1977) and women (Prudham
and Evans, 1981). The significance of this decline in prevalence rates
among the very elderly is not clear since the numbers of persons involved is
rather small, but it has been suggested that this may represent the survival
of an exceptionally fit élite (Exton-Smith, 1977). It is worth noting,
however, that although at age 65–74 falls are twice as common in women as
in men the sex difference is much less in extreme old age. The overall
female:male ratio in community studies is approximately 2 to 1 or higher
(Lucht, 1971; Prudham and Evans, 1981), but within a residential home
the ratio is much lower and approaches unity (Gryfe, Amies and Ashley,
1977). Retrospective information obtained from elderly persons living at
home estimates the annual incidence of falls per 1000 elderly persons to be
about 500 (Wild, Nayak and Isaacs, 1981). A 5-year prospective study in an
institutional population found a higher overall rate of 668 falls per 1000
persons per year (Gryfe, Amies and Ashley, 1977).

INJURY RATE

A commonly observed feature is that injury rates are much lower than the overall prevalence of falls. Studies based on elderly persons seen in a hospital accident and emergency department following a fall show an injury rate of 14–19 per 1000 persons over the age of 60, per year (Lucht, 1971; Waller, 1978). Interestingly the rate of severe falls (that is, those resulting in fractures or soft tissue injuries requiring suturing) is much higher within the protected environment of an institution at 117 falls per 1000 residents per year (Gryfe, Amies and Ashley, 1977).

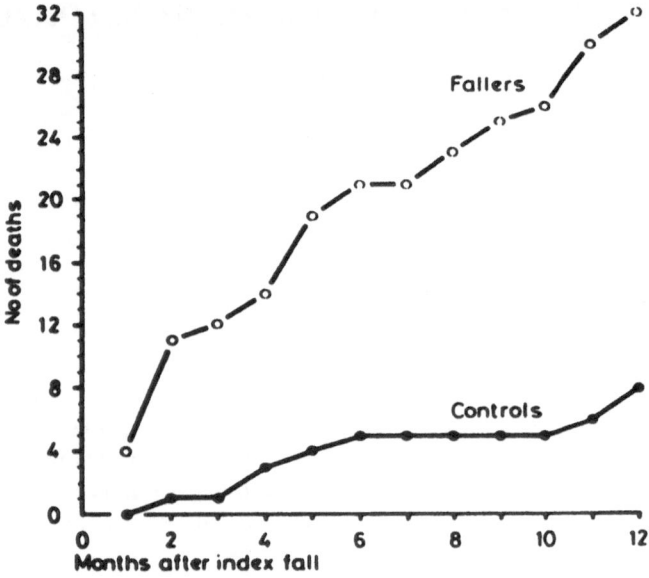

Figure 3.1   Cumulative mortality in 125 fallers and 125 controls in 12 months after index fall. (From Wild, Nayak and Isaacs, reproduced by permission of the editor of the *British Medical Journal*.)

MORTALITY

Old persons admitted to hospital because of a fall have a higher mortality than other patients in a geriatric unit (Naylor and Rosin, 1970). Of old persons who fall and injure themselves sufficiently to need the attention of their general practitioner or a hospital accident and emergency department 17–25% are dead within a year of the fall (Figure 3.1). In the great majority of cases the death does not appear to be related to the accident (Morfitt, 1983; Waller, 1978; Wild, Nayak and Isaacs, 1981). The number of fatal falls in the home rises with increasing age from 14.6 per 100 000 inhabitants for 65–74 years to 268.4 per 100 000 for 85 years and above

(Berfenstam, Lagerberg and Smedby, 1969). In the United States the death rate from falls for all ages has dropped from a high of about 19 per 100 000 in 1936 to less than nine per 100 000 in the early 1970s (Waller, 1974). There is a close relationship between mortality from falls and fractures of limbs, and deaths from falls appear to be positively associated with bone fragility (Eddy, 1978). Mortality is higher: among women than men and among white persons than non-white (Waller, 1974); in winter months (Lucht, 1971); in Scotland than in the south of England; and among urban compared with rural populations (Eddy, 1973). This is probably due to population differences in height since larger body size and greater height are associated with less bone loss with age.

ENVIRONMENTAL FACTORS

Typically, falls among elderly persons living at home occur indoors, usually in the living room or on the stairs (Clark, 1968; Lucht, 1971). Sheldon (1960) found that stairs accounted for one-third of all accidental falls. A frequent cause was missing the last step or the last group of steps in the mistaken belief that the bottom had been reached. U-shaped, two-flight stairs cause substantially fewer accidents than straight single flights and three-quarters of falls on stairs occur when the person is descending (Svanström, 1974). The majority of falls at home occur during the day (Lucht, 1971).

In institutions, however, the pattern of falls is different. The number of falls at night is higher, more falls occur when the person is actually in bed or a chair or attempting to get in or out of a bed or chair, and a high proportion of falls occur on the way to the toilet, perhaps as a result of hurrying due to the urgency of an unstable bladder (Gryfe, Amies and Ashley, 1977; Manjam and Mackinnon, 1973; Sehested and Severin-Nielsen, 1977). Patients most at risk are those accustomed to being active and independent and whose balance has been impaired by recent illness. Falls are more likely to occur during times of active rehabilitation although the serious injury rate is low. Paradoxically very low nursing staff levels are associated with a low fall rate because of reduced patient activity (Morris and Isaacs, 1980; Sehested and Severin-Nielsen, 1977). This became apparent during a period when the staff were taking industrial action, but whatever the cause of nurse staffing shortages the consequence tends to be that patients are kept in bed and are not encouraged to get out and walk. Unfortunately, the overzealous use of accident forms and quality assurance programmes, that investigate every fall no matter how trivial, tends to put nurses onto the defensive and may inhibit them from encouraging their patients to achieve full mobility. Optimum patient activity requires adequate numbers of nursing staff and occasional falls must be expected.

A hazardous environment has been blamed for up to one-third of all falls at home and the dangers of trailing wires, loose rugs, missing stair rods, polished floors, uneven pavements and poor lighting have been frequently pointed out (Agate, 1966; Gray, 1966; Sheldon, 1960). Waller (1978) has stressed the danger of walking aids, canes and wheelchairs. More recently, with the growing awareness of how frequently postural control is impaired in elderly persons, emphasis has centred less on environmental dangers and more on the underlying ill-health of fallers. Environmental factors are most relevant to fallers under the age of 75 years (Morfitt, 1983; Wild, Nayak and Isaacs, 1981).

DRUGS

In the United States 8% of falls causing injury have been attributed to alcohol. This usually occurs among persons who drink regularly and in large amounts (Waller, 1978). In the United Kingdom, however, fallers have not been found to differ from non-fallers in their consumption of alcohol (Prudham and Evans, 1981).

Falls have been linked to the consumption of hypnotics (Macdonald and Macdonald, 1977; Manjam and Mackinnon, 1973), but this association has not been found by others (Prudham and Evans, 1981; Sehested and Severin-Nielsen, 1977). However, fallers are more likely than non-fallers to be taking drugs particularly tranquillizers or diuretics (Campbell *et al.*, 1981; Prudham and Evans, 1981; Wild, Nayak and Isaacs, 1981). A 4-year prospective study found no evidence that antihypertensive medication increased the risk of falling (Stegman, 1983).

GAIT CHANGES IN FALLERS

Gait changes in elderly persons have been analysed using a variety of sophisticated electronic equipment (Imms and Edholm, 1979; Nayak *et al.*, 1982), but useful information has come from such simple methods as a stopwatch and measurement of the pattern left by ink-pads fixed to the heels of the subject's shoes. Using this technique Guimaraes and Isaacs (1980) studied the gait of four different groups: elderly patients who had been admitted to hospital shortly after a fall; patients of a similar age who had been admitted to hospital but who had not suffered a fall; normal active old people living at home who had fallen; normal active old people who had not fallen; controls were young normal subjects. Step length was longest in the young normal subjects (65 cm) and shortest in the hospital-ized fallers (22 cm). There was no difference between the step length of the non-hospitalized fallers and non-fallers, but hospitalized fallers had signi-ficantly shorter step lengths than hospitalized non-fallers. Speed of walking showed a similar pattern. The hospitalized fallers had a much greater range of frequency of stepping and their step length varied by 25% or more compared with less than 10% found in young normal subjects. Thus although the gait of normal old people showed some slowing of speed and shortening of step length the stride width and frequency of stepping were the same as in young controls and there was little variability in step length. No significant differences were found among active old people living at home regardless of whether or not they had fallen. Hospitalized non-fallers who were recovering from an acute illness walked slowly with short steps as if trying to maintain maximum stability. The group of hospitalized fallers, however, stood out because of their extremely short step length and slowness and their great variability of stepping frequency and step length. A quarter of these patients showed 'marche à petits pas' and were fearful of trying to walk lest they fell.

Demented elderly persons are more likely to fall than non-demented (Prudham and Evans, 1981; Wild, Nayak and Isaacs, 1981), and also have impaired gait compared with age-matched non-demented controls. Apparently normally ambulant demented subjects have significantly shorter step lengths, lower gait speed, lower stepping frequency, greater step-to-step variability, a greater double support ratio (that is, the ratio of time spent when both feet are on the ground to the total duration of the stride cycle) and a greater sway path (Visser, 1983).

NORMAL BALANCE

The upright standing body is not static but is maintained in that position by a dynamic process. One may think that one is standing completely still but, in fact, the body is making continuous adjustments in the sagittal plane. A vertical line through the centre of gravity lies on average a few centimetres in front of the transverse axis of the ankles, and slightly anterior to this line is the centre of pressure which is the centre of the distribution of the total force applied to the supporting surface (Murray, Seireg and Sepic, 1975). The upright position is maintained by active contraction of the calf muscles which keeps the vertical line through the centre of gravity behind the centre of pressure. This force of contraction of the muscles fluctuates continually at about 10 cycles/sec (Smith, 1957). Displacements of the body which threaten to shift the vertical line through the centre of gravity outside the support base are sensed by the eyes, vestibular apparatus and various proprioceptors. The information activates cerebral mechanisms, appropriate postural muscles contract and the vertical projection of the centre of gravity remains within the support base. In addition to this sway response, large displacing forces are corrected by stepping and hopping reactions or sweeping movements of the arms.

Postural sway has been measured by a variety of methods but one of the simplest ways is with the Wright ataxia meter (Wright, 1971) (since improved by Codoc Fabrications Limited). The subject stands with feet comfortably apart and the apparatus, which is contained within a small box, is placed on a table in front of the subject and connected by a thread to his/her waist. Sway is expressed as total angular movement in the anterior posterior plane only. A digital readout shows the degrees of arc

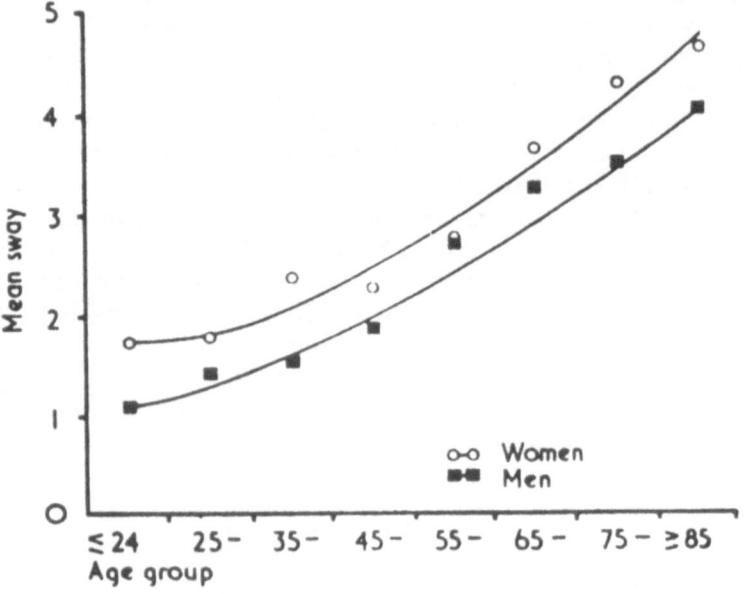

Figure 3.2 Regression of mean sway on age. (From Overstall *et al.*, 1977, reproduced by permission of the editor of the *British Medical Journal.*)

moved through in 1 min. Although force platforms and other more sophisticated equipment is available the ataxia meter is a convenient way of detecting disordered sensory motor function and in effect quantifies the Romberg test. In general, sway has been found to increase with advancing age (Figure 3.2) (Murray, Seireg, Sepic, 1975; Overstall *et al.*, 1977; Sheldon, 1963) but this age change is not so apparent within an institutional population (Fernie *et al.*, 1982). Loss of vibration sense but not impaired proprioception, vestibular function or visual acuity, is associated with increased sway in elderly subjects (Brocklehurst, Robertson and James-Groom, 1982).

Vision

It is generally found that closing the eyes increases postural sway and it appears that peripheral vision in particular is necessary for normal balance

(Begbie, 1967). Amputation above the knee only affects postural sway when the subject's eyes are closed indicating that the instability of the base and loss of proprioception is compensated for by increased dependence on vision (Fernie and Holliday, 1978). Similarly, patients with vestibular defects rely heavily on vision to maintain normal balance (Begbie, 1967; Martin, 1967).

It is not surprising therefore that Sheldon (1960) stressed the importance of inadequate illumination due either to defective vision or a fault in the actual lighting as a cause of falls. Although the number of falls that can be directly blamed on loss of visual cues is small, such as where the old person gets out of bed in the middle of the night without turning on the light and falls, it is likely that because of impairment in vestibular and proprioceptor systems even modest reductions in visual acuity can cause imbalance. Fractured femur patients aged 75 and over are less able to read small print than controls – a difficulty of which the patient is often unaware or regards as unimportant (Brocklehurst et al., 1976; Wilder-Smith and Thorp, 1981). There is, however, no difference between fallers and non-fallers in their use of spectacles (Prudham and Evans, 1981).

When fallers are compared with non-fallers they are found to have greater disturbance of visual perception of the vertical and horizontal. This was tested by asking patients to look at a rod on a video screen (Tobis, Nayak and Hoehler, 1981). The rod was rotated by the experimenter and the patient asked to identify when he/she thought it was vertical and when horizontal. Not only were the error scores higher in fallers, but were also higher in patients who had had a stroke with hemiplegia and in the very elderly. This finding of distorted visual perception supports two earlier reports on the role of vision in maintenance of balance. In 'moving room' experiments toddlers can be induced to fall forwards or backwards in the same direction as the surrounding 'room' moves. Presumably this is because the child's somatic proprioceptive information is poor since young adults do not fall but do sway more (Lee and Lishman, 1975). Over (1966) speculated that drop attacks occur because an unstable body position is induced by the false interpretation of visual stimulus and is not corrected by postural feedback. Where visual and postural information conflict women are found to be more 'field-dependent' than men; that is, they rely to a greater extent on the spatial framework provided by vision. If, as seems likely, the elderly come to rely more and more on vision to make up for defects in the other postural control systems, then falls could be induced by over-reliance on distorted visual perception.

Vestibular System

It appears that as one ascends the animal scale the vestibular system becomes less important (Magnus, 1926) and the information from eyes and proprioceptors and the system's central coordination is the essence of maintenance of normal balance. The vestibular mechanism plays no essential part in static posture or in the righting reactions; however, the vestibular system comes into action if the walking surface is uneven or the body is unstable (Martin, 1967).

LOSS OF POSTURAL REFLEXES AND FALLS

Although postural sway increases with age it is no higher in elderly persons who fall because of a trip or accident than in non-fallers of the same age. Trips and accidents account for about 45% of falls and the prevalence of this type of fall declines wth increasing age (Exton-Smith, 1977; Overstall et al., 1977; Sheldon, 1960). The general finding is that these accidental or 'environmental' falls are commoner under the age of 75 years and occur in relatively fit and mobile persons. They are more likely to get out of doors and expose themselves to the hazards of uneven pavements and icy steps, and their mortality is lower than that of spontaneous fallers (Campbell et al., 1981; Morfitt, 1983; Wild, Nayak and Isaacs, 1981).

Spontaneous fallers are those who fall because of drop attacks, loss of balance while standing or walking quietly or following a change of posture. Very often such patients can offer no explanation for their fall. Their postural sway is increased compared with age-matched non-fallers or accidental fallers (Overstall et al., 1977). Typically, these patients are over the age of 75 years, their gait and mobility are impaired and they are likely to be using a walking aid. Their mental test score and vision are also impaired, their functional ability is reduced and they need more support services and informal help (Campbell et al., 1981; Morfitt, 1983; Prudham and Evans, 1981).

Examination of these patients usually reveals multiple postural disabilities. The important proprioceptor information from cervical mechano-receptors is reduced by cervical spondylosis; vestibular function may be lost because of long-standing Ménière's disease; cataracts or glaucoma may have impaired vision; osteoarthritis of hips and lumbar spine may have reduced the normal suppleness and speed with which imbalance can be corrected; and Alzheimer's disease or cerebrovascular disease may have reduced the smooth cortical control of locomotion and balance. It is common to find patients with all these disabilities and it is not surprising therefore that one further insult, such as a chest infection, heart failure or a powerful hypnotic, can cause the person to fall. When examining the patient with falls it is important to assess each of these areas in turn so that the full level of disability can be gauged and appropriate treatment and rehabilitation planned.

DIZZINESS

Patients who blame their fall on dizziness or giddiness are found to have increased postural sway compared with controls (Overstall *et al.*, 1977); 7% of men and 6% of women under the age of 75 attribute their falls to dizziness compared with 20% of men and 16% of women aged 75 and over (Exton-Smith, 1977). These patients, therefore, are usually elderly, frail and often have obvious impairment of gait and balance. When one goes into their history it is found that only very rarely is true vertigo being described and more commonly the patients have a feeling of disequilibrium. Typically the sensation is provoked by movements of the body or head or in certain positions but not while otherwise remaining still (Orma and Koskenoja, 1957). Dizziness following head movements is commonly blamed on vertebrobasilar insufficiency but brain stem ischaemia is an uncommon finding in elderly patients investigated in a vestibular clinic (Overstall, Hazell and Johnson, 1981). Although true vertigo and drop attacks may follow transient ischaemia in the vertebrobasilar territory due to occlusion of the vertebral arteries by cervical osteophytes or emboli, this is relatively rare and the diagnosis is best avoided unless there is supporting evidence of brain stem dysfunction such as dysarthria, diplopia or homonomous hemianopia. Patients who complain of dizziness or disequilibrium after turning their head are more likely to have cervical mechanoreceptor dysfunction or a peripheral vestibular lesion or both.

Cervical Spondylosis

Cervical spondylosis affects nearly everyone over the age of 70 years, and whether it is a major factor in any particular patient's falls depends largely on the amount of compensation provided by other afferents into the postural control system. Cervical spondylosis is known to cause a variety of symptoms including attacks of vertigo, a constant feeling of unsteadiness during movements, nystagmus, deafness and tinnitus (Kuilman, 1959). The ataxia and vertigo particularly on head turning is due to an imbalance in the inflow of stimuli from damaged mechanoreceptors in the apophyseal joints of the cervical spine (Wyke, 1979). The activity from these receptors via extensive central connections exerts a powerful reflex influence on motor unit activity in the cervical and limb muscles and contributes significantly to postural and kinaesthetic sensation. Injecting local anaesthetic into the neck to interrupt the flow of afferent information from these joint receptors produces sensations that one often hears elderly fallers describe. There is a feeling of light-headedness and a sensation of being tilted and drawn towards the affected side 'like a bar of iron by a strong magnet' (de Jong *et al.*, 1977). Disturbed balance is also recognized as a feature of trauma to the second cervical spinal nerves (Behrmann, 1983). It is worth noting that immobilization of the neck in a cervical collar in patients who have cervical spondylosis often aggravates the feeling of disequilibrium particularly in the dark when the compensatory effects of vision are cancelled out. Cervical collars are therefore best avoided except for short-term relief of pain.

Vestibular Lesions

Two-thirds of elderly referrals to a vestibular clinic are found to have central vestibular lesions (most commonly the cerebellar syndrome), and one-third peripheral vestibular lesions (Overstall, Hazell and Johnson, 1981). The cerebellar syndrome is due to dysfunction of the cerebellar flocculus, nodulus and vermis, usually as a result of vascular insufficiency. Vertigo, especially where there is a rotatory sensation which persists when the eyes are closed indicates a vestibular lesion. Peripheral lesions are more likely than central ones to produce attacks of vertigo lasting hours or days, severe loss of balance and oscillopsia. The occurrence of drop attacks and other falls is about the same in both types of vestibular lesion. There is so much overlap between the two groups that the history is of little diagnostic help. A significant hearing loss and tinnitus is more common in a peripheral lesion but is not diagnostic. Factors that tend to point towards a diagnosis of a central vestibular lesion include poor eye tracking, fragmented or absent optokinetic nystagmus, positional nystagmus other than of the benign peripheral type and a very exaggerated caloric response (Hazell and Curotta, 1982). The precise diagnosis often depends on extensive testing but this is important for treatment. Peripheral lesions usually respond well to drugs and it is best to start initially with one of the antihistamines such as cinnarizine 15–30 mg three times a day; betahistine 8 mg three times a day is also effective treatment particularly for Ménière's disease. If no improvement is seen within 3 weeks there is little point in continuing the drug, and at this stage referral for specialist advice should be considered. Surgery (for example, decompression of the endolymphatic sac) for Ménière's disease is often helpful.

References

Agate, J. (1966). Accidents to old people in their homes. *Br. Med. J.*, **2**, 785–8.
Begbie, G. H. (1967). Some problems of postural sway. In de Reuck, A. V. S. and Knight, J. (eds.) *Myotic, Kinesthetic and Vestibular Mechanisms. Ciba Foundation Symposium*, pp. 80–92. (London: Churchill).
Behrman, S. (1983). Traumatic neuropathy of second cervical spinal nerve. *Br. Med. J.*, **286**, 1312–13.
Berfenstam, R., Lagerberg, D. and Smedby, B. (1969). Victim characteristics in fatal home accidents. *Acta Soc-med. Scand.*, **1**, 145–64.

Brocklehurst, J. C., Robertson, D. and James-Groom, P. (1982). Clinical correlates of sway in old age – sensory modalities. *Age Ageing*, **11**, 1–10.

Brocklehurst, J. C., Exton-Smith, A. N., Lempert Barber, S. M., Hunt, L. and Palmer, M. (1976). Fracture of the femur in old age; a two centre study of associated clinical factors and the cause of the fall. *Age Ageing*, **7**, 7–15.

Campbell, A. J., Reinken, J., Allan, B. C. and Martinez, G. S. (1981). Falls in old age; a study of frequency and related factors. *Age Ageing*, **10**, 264–70.

Clark, A. N. G. (1968). Factors in fracture of the female femur. *Geront. Clin.*, **10**, 257–70

de Jong, P. T. V. M., de Jong, J. M. B. V., Cohen, B. and Jongkees, L. B. W. (1977). Ataxia and nystagmus induced by injection of local anaesthetic in the neck. *Ann. Neurol.*, **1**, 240–6.

Eddy, T. P. (1973). Deaths from falls and fractures: comparison of mortality in Scotland and the United States with that in England and Wales. *Br. J. Prev. Soc. Med.*, **27**, 247–53.

Eddy, T. P. (1978). Falls and femoral fractures. *Br. Med. J.*, **2**, 955.

Exton-Smith, A. N. (1977). Functional consequences of ageing: clinical manifestations. In Exton-Smith, A. N. and Evans, J. G. (eds.) *Care of the Elderly: Meeting the Challenge of Dependency*, pp. 41–57. (London: Academic Press).

Fernie, G. R. and Holliday, P. J. (1978). Postural sway in amputees and normal subjects. *J. Bone Joint Surg.*, **60A**, 895–8.

Fernie, G. R., Gryfe, C. I., Holliday, P. J. and Llewellyn, A. (1982). The relationship of postural sway in standing to the incidence of falls in geriatric subjects. *Age Ageing*, **11**, 11–16.

Gray, B. (1966). *Home Accidents Among Older People.* (London: Royal Society for the Prevention of Accidents).

Gryfe, C. I., Amies, A. and Ashley, M. J. (1977). A longitudinal study of falls in an elderly population. 1. Incidence and morbidity. *Age Ageing*, **6**, 201–11.

Guimaraes, R. M. and Isaacs, B. (1980). Characteristics of the gait in old people who fall. *Int. Rehab. Med.*, **2**, 177–80.

Hazell, J. W. P. and Curotta, J. H. (1982). Vestibular disease in the elderly. In Sarner, M. (ed.) *Advanced Medicine 18*, pp. 238–249. (London: Pitman).

Imms, F. J. and Edholm, O. G. (1979). The assessment of gait and mobility in the elderly. *Age Ageing*, **8**, 261–7.

Kuilman, J. (1959). The importance of the cervical syndrome in otorhinolaryngology. *Prac. Otorhinolaryngol.*, **21**, 174–85.

Lee, D. and Lishman, R. (1975). Vision in movement and balance. *New Sci.*, **65**, 59.

Lucht, U. (1971). A prospective study of accidental falls and resulting injuries in the home among elderly people. *Acta Soc.-med. Scand.*, **2**, 105–20.

Macdonald, J. B. and Macdonald, E. T. (1977). Nocturnal femoral fracture and continuing widespread use of barbiturate hypnotics. *Br. Med. J.*, **2**, 483–5.

Magnus, R. (1926). Some results of studies in the physiology of posture. *Lancet*, **2**, 531 and 585.

Manjam, N. V. B. and Mackinnon, H. H. (1973). Patient, bed and bathroom. *Nova Scotia Med. Bull.*, **52**, 23–7.

Martin, J. P. (1967). Role of the vestibular system in the control of posture and movement in man. In de Reuck, A. V. S. and Knight, J. (eds.) *Myotic, Kinesthetic and Vestibular Mechanisms. Ciba Foundation Symposium*, pp. 92–96. (London: Churchill).

Morfitt, J. M. (1983). Falls in old people at home: intrinsic versus environmental factors in causation. *Pub. Hlth (London)*, **97**, 115–120.

Morris, E. V. and Isaacs, B. (1980). The prevention of falls in a geriatric hospital. *Age Ageing*, **9**, 181–5.

Murray, M. P., Seireg, A. A. and Sepic, S. B. (1975). Normal postural stability and steadiness: quantitative assessment. *J. Bone Joint Surg.*, **57A**, 510–16.

Nayak, U. S. L., Gabell, A., Simons, M. A. and Isaacs, B. (1982). Measurement of gait and balance in the elderly. *J. Am. Ger. Soc.*, **30**, 516–20.

Naylor, R. and Rosin, A. J. (1970). Falling as a cause of admission to a geriatric unit. *Practitioner*, **205**, 327–330.

Orma, E. J. and Koskenoja, M. (1957). Dizziness attacks and continuous dizziness in the aged. *Geriatrics*, **Feb.**, 92–100.

Over, R. (1966). Possible visual factors in falls by old people. *Gerontologist*, **6**, 212–14.

Overstall, P. W., Hazell, J. W. P. and Johnson, A. L. (1981). Vertigo in the elderly. *Age Ageing*, **10**, 105–9.

Overstall, P. W., Exton-Smith, A. N., Imms, F. J. and Johnson, A. L. (1977). Falls in the elderly related to postural imbalance. *Br. Med. J.*, **1**, 261–4.

Prudham, D. and Evans, J. G. (1981). Factors associated with falls in the elderly: a community study. *Age Ageing*, **10**, 141–6.

Sehested, P. and Severin-Nielsen, T. (1977). Falls by hospitalized elderly patients: causes, prevention. *Geriatrics*, **April**, 101–8.

Sheldon, J. H. (1948). *The Social Medicine of Old Age*. (London: Oxford University Press).

Sheldon, J. H. (1960). On the natural history of falls in old age. *Br. Med. J.*, **2**, 1685–90.

Sheldon, J. H. (1963). The effect of age on the control of sway. *Geront. Clin.*, **5**, 129–38.

Smith, J. W. (1957). The forces operating at the human ankle joint during standing. *J. Anat.*, **91**, 545–64.

Stegman, M. R. (1983). Falls among elderly hypertensives – are they iatrogenic? *Gerontology*, **29**, 399–406.

Svanström, L. (1974). Falls on stairs: an epidemiological accident study. *Scand. J. Soc. Med.*, **2**, 113–20.

Tobis, J. S., Nayak, U. S. L. and Hoehler, F. (1981). Visual perception of verticality and horizontality among elderly fallers. *Arch. Phys. Med. Rehabil.*, **62**, 619–22.

Visser, H. (1983). Gait and balance in senile dementia of Alzheimer's type. *Age Ageing*, **12**, 296–301.

Waller, J. A. (1974). Injury in aged. *NY State J. Med.*, **74**, 2200–8.

Waller, J. A. (1978). Falls among the elderly – human and environmental factors. *Accid. Anal. Prev.*, **10**, 21–33.

Wild, D., Nayak, U. S. L. and Isaacs, B. (1981). How dangerous are falls in old people at home? *Br. Med. J.*, **282**, 2132–3.

Wright, B. M. (1971). A simple mechanical ataxiameter. *J. Physiol.*, **218**, 27–8P.

Wilder-Smith, O. H. G. and Thorp, T. A. S. (1981). How dangerous are falls in old people at home? *Br. Med. J.*, **282**, 2132–3.

Wyke, B. (1979). Cervical articular contributions to posture and gait: their relations to senile disequilibrium. *Age Ageing*, **8**, 251–8.

4

Falls in Old Age: Clinical Aspects

A. J. D. FARQUHARSON

INTRODUCTION

The occurrence of a fall involving an elderly person commonly confronts the physician with a diagnostic problem of considerable difficulty. It is, moreover, in practice a not infrequent challenge, as previous sections of this book discuss in detail (pp. 15–26).

The clinical exercise begins with an attempt to establish whether the fall was due to an accident such as a trip, slip, stumble, etc. which might be expected to result in a fall at any age. Even if the available evidence points to the fall being accidental in nature, the wise physician is aware of other factors which might contribute to such a fall. Conditions such as dementia, intoxication and defective vision are all likely to lead to the occurrence of falls and other mishaps.

PATHOLOGICAL FALLS

Accidental falls, however, rarely recur even in the elderly, therefore the patient with repeated falls almost certainly has a major pathological factor contributing to the presentation. In particular falls out of bed are nearly always pathological in nature and usually signify a poor prognosis.

Falls that occur without an obvious environmental cause are, therefore, likely to be due to a major dysfunction in one or more parts of the systems that control posture and balance. The human body has been likened to an antigravity machine that is in constant danger of breaking down. It follows that as failure of any part of the machine is likely to lead to a violent and damaging contact with terra firma, so the diagnostic exercise may have to embrace the very wide body of general medicine. Such falls can be regarded as *pathological* or 'pattern' falls.

Pathological falls may be divided into two main groups by the answer to a simple question. Was the event associated with loss of consciousness? If the answer to the question is in the affirmative then the diagnosis must be one of the causes of syncope or epilepsy.

EPILEPSY

Epilepsy is common in the elderly; in about two-thirds of cases it is generalized in type, the remainder being composed of various degrees of partial seizures. The diagnosis depends initially on an eye-witness account of the phenomenon, a previous history of fits and sometimes an account of a warning or aura by the patient. Other circumstances of the case that raise the suspicion of epilepsy are incontinence during an attack and the production of unexplained injuries.

An epileptic episode may be followed by post-ictal (Todd's) paresis which usually lasts less then 48 hours but has been known to continue for 4 days. In addition various degrees of post-ictal confusion, sometimes lasting as long as 7 days, may occur. The excellent papers by Roberts, Godfrey and Caird (1982) reveal that in their series of 81 elderly patients presenting with epilepsy, 16% suffered Todd's paresis and 14% a confusional state lasting 24 hours or more. Three patients had both types of post-ictal problems. It is obvious that it is not difficult to misdiagnose such cases as *transient ischaemic attacks,* but because of the differences in investigation, management and prognosis it is very important not so to do.

Clinical assessment of the elderly victim of a seizure must include a search for any cause outside the central nervous system such as hypoglycaemia, renal failure, epileptogenic drugs, hyperosmolar non-ketotic diabetic coma and hypocalcaemia amongst 'metabolic' conditions. Cardiovascular problems such as aortic stenosis, severe postural hypotension, left ventricular failure and possibly cardiac dysrhythmias may also provoke an epileptic phenomenon.

The commonest cause of seizures in the elderly is cerebral infarction; epilepsy may herald a stroke or occur many months afterwards. Cerebral tumours are the next most common cause (12% in Roberts *et al.*'s series). As in younger patients, epilepsy may reflect the presence of a subdural haematoma.

Epilepsy may, as is well known, be a sequel of head injury. It is perhaps less well known that seizures may arise *de novo* in dementia of Alzheimer type. Seizures of an apparently idiopathic nature may also first appear in old age.

Patients with seizures of recent origin and no obvious clinical cause merit investigation, particularly if there are focal neurological signs, the most useful investigations being electroencephalography, isotope brain scan (scintiscan), and CAT brain scan if either of the former are positive. Roberts and Caird, however, advise that a CAT scan is indicated only in the presence of a positive scintiscan or progressive focal neurological signs.

Finally, there is always the rare bird, such as the patient treated in my own unit, a widow of 73, who presented with three grand mal fits with increasing postictal confusion over a period of about 1 month. Investigation revealed the presence of positive serological tests for syphilis both in blood and cerebrospinal fluid. Treatment with penicillin has proved totally effective, there being no recurrence in 5 years.

Phenytoin

The treatment of the elderly epileptic usually presents no great problems, with the exception of many cases of poor compliance. Compliance, however, is likely to be improved by one daily dosage, usually at night, if phenytoin is the most suitable drug.

Partial seizures and tonic-clonic (grand mal) seizures usually respond well to phenytoin in a dose of 200–400 mg at night. Phenytoin has the additional advantage of the ready availability of serum level assay as a guide to dosage and compliance. The occurrence of nystagmus, ataxia and confusion is a toxic (overdosage) effect of phenytoin and not a side-effect.

Phenobarbitone and other Drugs

Phenobarbitone should not be used in the elderly as increased confusion, drowsiness or agitation are likely to result. Typical absences (petit mal) and atypical absences (atonic or akinetic seizures), usually respond to *sodium valproate* 1800 mg daily in divided doses. *Ethosuximide* may be useful in petit mal; *carbamazepine* can be used in the control of partial or grand mal seizures. *Combination therapy* should be avoided or used only as a last resort.

SYNCOPE

The causes of syncope are legion and often very difficult to determine especially when the patient is vague, confused, deaf or dysphasic. Nevertheless, the effort must be made to achieve an accurate diagnosis, because the prospects of effective treatment are, in many cases, excellent. As always, a good history is the key to rapid and accurate diagnosis.

A common cause is a simple or vasovagal faint provoked by emotional shock or unpleasant experiences or sights. Management consists of reassurance in such circumstances.

Micturition syncope is almost confined to the male sex and is managed well by advice to sit down to urinate! *Defaecation syncope* is very rare but probably best managed by the use of laxatives and the avoidance of straining at stool. Syncope occurring in the environment of the toilet, particularly in hospitalized patients, should alert the physician to the possibility of *pulmonary embolism*, a suspicion enhanced by the presence of evidence of venous thrombosis in the lower limbs and pelvis, tachypnoea, chest pain, haemoptysis and cardiographic evidence of right-sided heart strain. In cases of doubt a lung scintiscan may confirm the diagnosis. The treatment is prompt anticoagulation, for which there is no upper age limit, other factors permitting.

Cough syncope is another reflex form of faint, generally provoked by a sustained spasm of forceful coughing. Management depends on treating the cause of the cough, if possible.

Syncope has been described in association with swallowing due to a variety of *oesophageal conditions*, such as diverticulum. Anticholinergic drugs may be effective in controlling the symptoms. Syncope and pain occurring on swallowing may be due to *glossopharyngeal neuralgia* for which the treatment is carbamazepine or neural block.

Cervical Spondylosis and Carotid Sinus Sensitivity

Faintness, giddiness and syncope are commonly associated with neck movements in the elderly. It is important to differentiate between neck movements and head movements, as changes in head position may provoke symptoms due to labyrinthine and other disorders. If the symptoms are induced by neck movements by far the likeliest cause is the presence of cervical spondylosis, particularly if other features of vertebrobasilar ischaemia, such as true vertigo, diplopia, amblyopia, dysarthria and sensory changes in the face, are present. So many elderly people have radiographic evidence of apparently severe cervical spondylosis, but remain asymptomatic, that unless there are clear indications of vertebrobasilar ischaemia in association with movement of the neck, the diagnosis cannot with certainty be ascribed to the condition of the joints in the cervical spine.

Another but quite unusual cause of syncope on neck turning is carotid sinus sensitivity. In this condition carotid sinus massage will provoke the symptoms. If simple advice such as the avoidance of rapid or extreme neck movements, and the prohibition of tight collars, cravats, etc., fails to relieve the symptoms, a permanent cardiac demand pacemaker is usually highly effective.

However, in elderly patients, cervical spondylosis is by far the commonest problem. The sufferers can be helped by advice to reduce neck movements, a cervical collar and non-steroidal anti-inflammatory medication usually in that order of priority.

Aortic Stenosis

Occasionally a patient is seen in which syncope is clearly related to effort. In most of such cases the problem is located in the outflow tract of the left ventricle. In the vast majority of cases aortic stenosis is present. Usually this implies a very severe degree of stenosis requiring expert cardiological assessment and treatment.

Much rarer causes of outflow tract obstruction of the left ventricle are the various forms of subaortic stenosis, hypertrophic cardiomyopathy; left atrial thrombi and pedunculated atrial myxomas occasionally impact in the mitral valve.

Exercise electrocardiography may reveal a dysrhythmia provoked by effort and amenable to treatment.

POSTURAL HYPOTENSION

Many elderly patients complain of dizziness and some even faint on standing up from bed or chair. Some of these patients have a clinically demonstrable drop in systolic blood pressure on standing. Postural or orthostatic hypotension is present by definition when systolic pressure drops by 20 mmHg or more after standing for 2 min.

The whole subject of postural hypotension is, however, far from straightforward.

Many old people have postural hypotension – 24% in one survey (Caird, Andrews and Kennedy, 1973), but few have symptoms, presumably due to the presence of intact autoregulation of cerebral blood flow. Cerebral perfusion is protected in normality from variations in systolic blood pressure, by an intrinsic regulatory system which ensures an even blood flow through the brain over a wide range of perfusion pressure.

As already suggested, many old people feel faint on rising to their feet who do not have postural hypotension. However, if the patient has typical symptoms and has postural hypotension then it is not unreasonable to assume a connection!

Medication in Postural Hypotension

In my experience a common cause of symptomatic postural hypotension in the elderly is medication. The most severe problems are seen with antihypertensive agents, esepcially those with a peripheral action.

Other drugs likely to be responsible are diuretics, phenothiazines, barbiturates, benzodiazapines, digoxin and levodopa.

Other Causes

If evidence of autonomic dysfunction is present, such as lack of sweating, absence of reflex tachycardia on standing and loss of sinus arrhythmia, then the presence of neurological conditions such as neurosyphilis, diabetic neuropathy, Parkinson's disease. Wernicke's encephalopathy and Shy–Drager syndrome might be suspected.

Postural hypotension occurs in states of hypovolaemia due to any cause, for example, blood loss, inadequate fluid intake, Addison's disease, etc., but in most cases in the elderly of syncope and postural hypotension no obvious aetiology is found. There is some evidence that the main aetiological factor in postural hypotension in the elderly is the increasing arterial and arteriolar rigidity in this age group (Maclennan, Hall and Timothy, 1980).

Management consists in treating any underlying condition, and altering the prescription sheet if indicated. For idiopathic cases, the symptoms can often be controlled by advice of the 'get up slowly' type, and by the use of supportive hose or bandaging of the lower limbs. Mineralocorticoids have been used but, except in the case of Addison's disease, generally prove to be of little help to the elderly patient.

HYPOGLYCAEMIA

Hypoglycaemia is an important cause of loss of consciousness, a diagnosis suggested by treatment for diabetes, delirium, sweating and hunger. A glucose tolerance test followed by fasting may suggest the presence of *reactive hypoglycaemia*, especially following gastroduodenal surgery or small bowel resection etc., or the existence of an *insulinoma*.

It should be remembered that hypoglycaemia due to oral agents particularly chlorpropamide, may be prolonged and recur many hours after initial treatment with glucose. Hypoglycaemia may also present as epilepsy or with focal neurological signs such as hemiparesis.

CARDIAC SYNCOPE

Cardiac syncope may be suggested by the observation of flushing after an attack or the presence of palpitations or sudden onset of chest pain, dyspnoea or cyanosis. There is no doubt that Stokes–Adams attacks are responsible for syncope as may be other conditions in group I of Jonas' classification (Jonas, Klein and Dimant, 1977), that is SVT longer than 6 sec and of 150 beats/min or more,

or, VT > 6 sec > 120 bpm
or, Bradycardia > 6 sec and less than 40 bpm
or, Asystole 4 sec or more in duration.

The correlation between many other degrees and types of arrhythmias and syncope or faintness is, however, not very strong.

It is now well known that many asymptomatic old people have ECG abnormalities demonstrable by ambulatory electrocardiography (Rai, 1982; Taylor and Stout, 1983), which on follow-up do not cause increased morbidity or mortality.

The ascribing of syncope and other symptoms to ECG abnormalities must, therefore, be made with great caution. It is even doubtful if 24 hour ambulatory electrocardiography is helpful in the diagnosis of syncope, despite which I certainly have seen several cases when the investigation did result in effective treatment.

I will not dwell on the treatment of various dysrhythmias except to say that the older and well-established drugs should be used in the first instance. The elderly tolerate cardiac pacing well, although in the United Kingdom this procedure is not generally used for asymptomatic idioventricular rhythm or partial degrees of heart block.

Acute Myocardial Infarction

It should be noted that acute myocardial infarction quite often presents as syncope alone. Hospital-based studies have shown the incidence, as a percentage of all infarction cases, to be between 5 and 12%.

It would thus seem to be the case that unless syncope is clearly due to some definite non-cardiac cause, thorough examination of the heart including ECG is essential in the investigation of syncope, faintness and falls of the elderly subjects.

Routine biochemical screening as well as indicating hypoglycaemia may be useful in revealing hypokalaemia which may in association with digoxin result in a severe tachycardia.

Hypocalcaemia and Hyperventilation

Hypocalcaemia may also be uncovered and lead to a diagnosis of vitamin D deficiency, malabsorption or hypoparathyroidism. The classical symptoms

of hypocalcaemia are tingling and numbness in the fingers, toes and in the
face.

The last condition I will mention under the heading of syncope as a cause
of falls is 'hysterical' *hyperventilation* which usually the subject is only too
willing to demonstrate, and which when all is considered is much more
common than many of the conditions previously discussed.

BRAIN FAILURE AND FALLS

Prudham and Evans' (1981) study of factors associated with falls, showed
that where there was a history of a fall in the previous 12 months, 32.6%
reported the occurrence of a faint or blackout, 47.5% reported vertigo,
35.7% reported episodes of weakness, or numbness and 22.8% reported
episodes of double vision. A significantly higher proportion of fallers than
non-fallers also appeared to have an impaired mental test score.

It is thus apparent that many pathological falls in the elderly are
associated with factors other than syncope or epilepsy. It is recognized that
the incidence of significant *dementia* is very common in the old (20% over
the age of 80). Another way of looking at dementia is to think of it as a
cause of *chronic brain failure.* There is evidence (Visser, 1983) of widespread deterioration of gait in dementia, even in apparently normally
ambulant subjects. It is not surprising then that it is a matter of common
clinical experience that many elderly 'fallers' are confused, disorientated
and incontinent. These unfortunate old people represent a medical
emergency because of the possibility of the presence of *acute, or acute on
chronic, brain failure*, as the cause of the fall and the clinical presentation.
The vital component of the central nervous system is, of course, the
neurone, regarding which three salient facts must always be remembered:

1. Neurones will function normally only within narrow limits of environmental conditions.
2. If the above limits are exceeded greatly or for any length of time, for
   example anoxia for 4 min, neurones will begin to die in large
   numbers.
3. Neurones are incapable of mitotic division and, therefore, cannot be
   replaced.

It follows then that any deviation from normality in the environment of
the neurone must be detected and treated with great urgency if further
permanent brain damage is not to ensue.

I will now consider some of the common disturbances of the *milieu
intérieur* which so frequently afflict the elderly patient causing acute
derangement of function of the central nervous system. The first step in
management is to try to establish whether the condition is acute or chronic.

If it appears the patient was independent, self-caring, cooking, shopping, etc., until a few days or even a week or two before the onset of the present highly dependent state, then it is obvious that an acute condition is present. On the other hand, if there is a long history of memory loss, disorientation, self-neglect, poor gait and incontinence, then the problem is undeniably chronic. In case of doubt, it is wise to assume the problem is one of acute brain failure.

The commonest causes of acute or acute on chronic brain failure are generally multiple; for example, the confused, disorientated patient who has fallen may well be found to have: bronchopneumonia with, in the very old, few clinical signs, little cough, no sputum and often no pyrexia; which has led in combination with right-sided heart failure to cerebral hypoxia; owing to immobility and inanition fluid intake is likely to have been low over the preceding few days and dehydration is present; in addition, it is only too probable that because of increasing restlessness and confusion a sedative or hypnotic drug will have been prescribed; the clinical picture may be further complicated by the presence of injuries sustained in the fall with resultant pain, shock, blood loss, etc.

The above is, I consider, not an untypical example of an elderly 'social problem' so often referred to geriatric departments for 'further care', who is in fact suffering from nine or more eminently treatable conditions.

Influences on Possible Brain Failure

I will not dwell on every cause of acute brain failure at length as this subject would merit an entire volume if not a series on its own. It would, however, be helpful to the physician or surgeon confronted with such a problem to bear the following list of malign cerebral influences in mind:

1. any cause of alteration of blood gases – *hypoxia*, CO_2 narcosis, oxygen intoxication, carbon dioxide poisoning;
2. any cause of hypovolaemia – *dehydration*, blood loss, overprescription of diuretics, etc. – because of impaired renal function the elderly are particularly liable to the rapid development of severe dehydration;
3. alteration of body temperature – *pyrexia* and *hypothermia*.
4. any cause of extremes of blood pressure – *hypotension*, cardiac disasters, blood loss and drugs and severe or malignant hypertension;
5. *raised intracranial pressure* – cerebral oedema, cerebrovascular accident, tumour, subdural haematoma, etc.;
6. any alteration in plasma electrolytes or pH, especially *hypercalcaemia* but also hypokalaemia, hyponatraemia, *uraemia* and non-ketotic hyperosmolar diabetic coma;

7. any alteration in blood glucose – *hypoglycaemia* and hyper-glycaemia;

8. *metabolic disorders* – thyroid, adrenal, parathyroid and pituitary malfunction;

9. intoxication with *alcohol* or *drugs* – especially sedatives, tranquil-lizers, anticonvulsants, levodopa, antidepressants, anticholinergics, beta-blockers, methyldopa, reserpines and major narcotics.

   The same week that a leading article was published in the *British Medical Journal* (Szabadi, 1984), I saw an elderly man at home who had been prescribed tablets of chlorpromazine 100 mg t.d.s., loving-ly administered over a 2-week period by his sister, a retired nurse. As a result the patient had developed a *neuroleptic malignant syndrome*. This patient exhibited the motor group of symptoms. He was pale, stuporose, akinetic and mute, but there were no extra-pyramidal features (rigidity, bradykinesia, tremor, chorea and oculogyric crisis), or autonomic complications (hyperpyrexia, blood pressure and heart rate variations, etc.). This patient recovered completely and was discharged from hospital apparently fit and well some 7 days after admission;

10. avitaminoses, especially B_{12} and B_1 (thiamine) deficiency. The Wernicke/Korsakoff syndrome is due to vitamin B_1 deficiency, usually but not always associated with alcoholism, but it may also develop in the undernourished or as a consequence of malabsorp-tion. Wernicke's encephalopathy is characterized by ataxia, peripheral neuropathy and postural hypotension. A disorder of gaze, usually nystagmus, is present in practically every case. This condition (Wernicke's) is probably much underdiagnosed. In an article in the *British Medical Journal* (1969), it was stated that only four cases had been seen at post mortem in 21 years. But Harper (1979) reported on the necropsy of 51 cases seen in only 4 years, of which only seven had been diagnosed in life. Treatment with vitamin B_1 – the most convenient preparation is Parentrovite – is usually highly effective as far as the motor and peripheral nervous systems are concerned. Unfortunately, the associated dementia and psych-osis (Korsakoff's syndrome) does not respond so well;

11. infections of the central nervous system such as meningitis (unusual but not rare), neurosyphilis (now rare), and encephalitis, must be remembered. Elderly persons are particularly prone to eruptions of herpes zoster. The eruption is often accompanied by the develop-ment of a *zoster encephalitis* the features of which are drowsiness, sometimes progressing to stupor, confusion, anorexia and profound weakness. The prognosis is usually excellent provided that good nurs-ing care is available to avoid the complications of dehydration, hypo-static pneumonia and decubitus ulcers;

12. in all cases of acute brain failure when the diagnosis cannot be fully justified by the presence of other conditions, septicaemia and subacute bacterial endocarditis must be excluded. In all such cases serial blood cultures are mandatory.

TRANSIENT ISCHAEMIC ATTACKS (TIAs)

Transient ischaemic attacks (TIA's) are a common cause of falls in the elderly; they are even more commonly misdiagnosed as drop attacks or epilepsy. This problem in diagnosis is not surprising as all three of the above conditions may present in the same patient, and indeed may all be due to a common cause – cerebrovascular disease.

The typical transient ischaemic attack presents with the sudden onset of weakness and/or altered sensation in one or more limbs or parts of the body. Transient monocular blindness (amaurosis fugax), or varying degrees of hemianopia may occur. Hemianopia may occur with vertigo due to vertebrobasilar involvement, or vertigo may be the sole symptom. Syncope may be associated with transient ischaemic attacks which affect the brainstem.

Whatever the symptoms and signs the duration is brief, often only a few minutes; less commonly the condition lasts a few hours, signs and symptoms gradually improving over the duration of the attack.

Suspicion that the disturbance may be due to a transient ischaemic attack is heightened by the finding on examination of the heart and carotid vessels of a possible source of emboli, such as carotid bruits, aortic systolic murmurs, atrial fibrillation, mitral stenosis, mitral valve prolapse, evidence of a recent myocardial infarction, left atrial myxoma, subacute bacterial endocarditis, etc.

The importance of transient ischaemic attacks is, of course, the prognostic significance – there appears to be an approximate 60% risk of developing a stroke within 5 years of presenting with a transient ischaemic attack.

Treatment of the elderly patient usually consists of drugs that inhibit platelet function, such as aspirin and dipyridamole. There is some recent evidence that combination therapy may be more effective than either drug prescribed alone. However, although most trials indicate that aspirin is of some benefit, the results are inconsistent, probably because transient ischaemic attacks are a symptom complex with several causes. It seems reasonable at present to treat vertebrobasilar and transient ischaemic attacks of brief duration with an antiplatelet agent such as aspirin. Those of longer duration, that is those lasting 30 min or more, are more likely to be due to thrombotic emboli and are, therefore, more likely to be controlled by anticoagulant treatment.

In all cases, careful consideration should be given to direct treatment of the underlying cause, that is, carotid artery or heart valve surgery. Such a decision, however, can only be reached after extensive specialized investigation the discussion of which is beyond the scope of the present writing.

DROP ATTACKS

A common presentation of a fall in old age is that the victim will say 'I was just standing at the sink (or at the bus stop or walking across the room, etc.) when my legs gave way and down I went!' It will be noted that there was no warning, no loss of consciousness and no report of vertigo. Many of the patients thus afflicted once having fallen are unable to rise unaided but, with help, once raised to their feet are able to stand and walk normally. This describes a typical drop attack. Drop attacks are common and are responsible for 12–25% of falls in the elderly (Overstall et al., 1977; Sheldon, 1960). The great majority of sufferers are women, and attacks tend to be recurrent and unpredictable.

The defect responsible for drop attacks is still a matter for debate. Although there is no doubt that vertebrobasilar ischaemia can cause the phenomenon, most of the patients seen in practice have no history of vertigo, visual disturbance or disorder of facial sensation, etc., which would indicate problems in the brain stem. The most attractive hypothesis is that put forward by Overstall (1978) postulating that 'drop attacks occur because an unstable body position is induced by the false interpretation of visual stimulation and is not corrected by postural feedback'.

Considering the large numbers of elderly people with visual problems and the almost universal decline in proprioception, as measured by loss of ankle jerks and impaired vibration sensation in the lower limbs, in an ageing population it is not surprising, if the hypotheses were to be confirmed, that drop attacks are so common. The postulation would also to a large extent explain the frequently observed 'grabbing granny' who navigates about the home from one article of furniture to another and then to the wall, etc. It will be noticed by the observant that the object is 'grabbed' not for support but probably for steadiness or, to use nautical jargon, a 'position fix' in an otherwise dimly perceived environment.

There is, therefore, scope for treatment to help some of these cases. Cervical spondylosis and vertebrobasilar ischaemia may be treated as outlined earlier. In other cases treatable causes of visual impairment, peripheral neuropathy or proprioceptive loss (B_{12} deficiency, tabes dorsalis) should be sought. The provision of a walking aid such as a frame or stick may help some cases, the problem being, of course, that when the aid is moved the patient is once again reliant on a defective antigravity system. This can be overcome to some extent by the use of a 'rolator' type of walking frame, which usually works well in institutions, but is often too bulky and unwieldy to be of practical use in the frequently small and furniture-cluttered rooms of the elderly at home.

Dizziness

Old people who fall complain frequently of dizziness or vertigo. Dizziness is an ill-defined complaint, often made to describe a sensation of unsteadiness or imbalance in the lower limbs as 'No I don't feel as if things are going round doctor, I just feel shaky on my legs'. Such a patient should be examined carefully for evidence of neurological problems such as cerebellar ataxia, monoplegia or paraplegia, proprioceptive loss or some form of muscular weakness. As always much information can be obtained from the observation of gait, and thus with no equipment other than a tendon hammer and a tuning fork, one may diagnose yet another 'social problem'!

Cerebellar ataxia in the elderly may be due to stroke (abrupt onset), degenerative process (slowly progressive) or malignant disease, primary, secondary or non-metastatic (usually rapidly progressive). Many sufferers from *multiple sclerosis* survive into old age presenting with a variety of symptoms amongst which an ataxia is usually prominent.

Special care should be taken to exclude *spinal cord lesions* particularly tumours which, in the early and treatable stage, may present with no more than unsteadiness in the legs and falls.

Dizziness and falls may also be due to *muscular weakness* commonly due to hypokalaemia, osteomalacia, malignant cachexia, polymyositis or polymyopathy due to diabetes, steroid therapy (or Cushing's syndrome); hypothyroidism (myxoedematous myopathy); myasthenia gravis or myasthenic syndrome (?underlying bronchogenic cancer); sufferers from dystrophia myotonica and Charcot–Marie–Tooth dystrophy often survive into old age, occasionally undiagnosed (or more likely the diagnosis has long since been forgotten!).

Motor neurone disease is frequently seen or, in my experience, not seen and misdiagnosed. The syndrome as seen in the elderly of profound widespread weakness and weight loss of a progressive nature often results in a fruitless search for underlying malignant disease. The diagnosis, once thought of, is usually easily made by the finding of fibrillation, wasting and paresis of the tongue.

Dizziness is a term often used by patients to describe a muzziness or 'fuzzy feeling' in the head, the causes of which are legion but usually systemic in nature such as anaemia, cardiac failure, renal failure, etc. One of the common causes of this symptom is the effect of medication, particularly sedatives, tranquillizers and anticonvulsants. Many other drugs, however, can cause the symptom. Due to impaired renal function in old age, amongst other factors, metabolism of many drugs is delayed, resulting in high tissue levels. For this reason, where possible, drugs with a short half-life should be preferred, and those with a very long half-life, such as nitrazepam or flurazepam, avoided.

Some drugs are, of course, *ototoxic* and may produce a sensation of vertigo or dizziness; they include: aminoglycosides, anti-inflammatory agents, frusemide, ethacrynic acid, salicylates, quinine, chloroquinine and chlordiazepoxide.

Dizziness may also be the complaint in a number of subjects already discussed above, including postural hypotension, transient ischaemic attacks, epilepsy, cervical spondylosis, cardiac dysrhythmias, hypoglycaemia, etc.

Psychiatric disorders often have dizziness amongst their symptoms, but such patients rarely fall except as a result of drugs or hysteria. However, even the lifelong sufferer from chronic anxiety must one day pass through the gate between life and death usually because of organic disease, which fact must always be borne in mind in the management of such a patient.

Vertigo

Dizziness and vertigo are often confused, but once again the taking of an accurate history is of vital importance, as true vertigo indicates a vestibular dysfunction. Vertigo involves the sensation of rotation either of the patient or the environment. Vertigo is frequently associated with other disturbances such as nausea, vomiting, pallor and sweating particularly if the onset is acute – as in motion sickness.

Middle ear disease as evidenced by discharge, perforation and conductive hearing loss, may result in infection spreading to the labyrinth, which if suspected demands full specialist assessment.

Sensorineural deafness and vertigo suggest the presence of *Ménière's disease* if the symptoms are intermittent and particularly if there is associated nausea, vomiting and tinnitus. This is a frequently over-diagnosed condition in the elderly, many of whom are thereby sentenced to lifelong treatment with antihistamines or phenothiazines. As the diagnosis can be made with some accuracy merely by taking a history and with the use of a tuning fork, there is little excuse for such incompetent management.

If sensorineural deafness is unilateral and progressive, a search should be made for seventh cranial nerve damage, that is, facial paresis, and loss of corneal reflex. The presence of cerebellar signs also suggest the presence of an *acoustic neuroma* or other cerebellopontine angle lesion. A CAT scan and a neurosurgical opinion are usually indicated. In one of my patients who complained of vertigo it was discovered that the mould of his hearing aid was too large for the external auditory canal.

Vertigo occurring without deafness, but with focal neurological signs usually indicates, in older patients, an ischaemic or neoplastic lesion. Multiple sclerosis is occasionally seen *de novo* in the middle-aged. In younger persons basilar migraine should be considered.

Vertigo presenting without deafness or focal neurological signs is due either to *acute labyrinthitis*, the cause of which is unknown, possibly viral, and the course is benign; or to *benign positional vertigo* in which the symptom is induced by changes in *head* position. This condition may be tested for as follows:

1. The patient sits upright on couch.
2. Patient is instructed to fix gaze on examiner's forehead.
3. The patient's head is then rotated through 45° and lowered at the same time to 30° below horizontal beyond the end of the couch.
4. The head is then rotated through 90° to the other side.
5. The examiner looks for nystagmus. Providing the patient is fit and cooperative there are two positive responses. The commonest response is the development of severe vertigo and nystagmus towards the lower ear; after a short latent period the symptoms last for about 30 s then abate. Repeated testing shows adaptation with a diminished response. This response indicates *benign positional vertigo*. The other response that may occur is the development with no latent period of nystagmus, with no vertigo. The nystagmus does not abate and there is no adaptation. This second response usually indicates a *posterior fossa tumour*, or occasionally a vascular lesion or multiple sclerosis.

Benign positional vertigo is of limited duration and may be helped by Cawthorne–Cooksey exercises as described by Finestone (1982).

Vertigo and/or dizziness may be a prolonged sequel of head injury especially in the elderly. Usually there are no focal signs and the condition gradually abates but may last many months or years.

CHRONIC DISABILITIES INVOLVING GAIT

Chronic disabilities involving gait may obviously lead to falls, frequently repeated. Prime amongst this group are the patients with advanced Parkinson's disease and other extrapyramidal syndromes. The gait is slow, shuffling and unstable, sufferers are most liable to trip over very small obstructions. In Parkinson's disease falls are likely to occur due to the development of complications such as postural hypotension or dementia. Treatment with levodopa or bromocriptine can result in falls due to the development of choreoathetoid dystonias, which are an indication to reduce the dose. The drugs must not be abruptly discontinued as the patient is likely to become severely disabled by rigidity and bradykinesia.

Hemiplegic and arthritic patients perhaps do not fall as often as one might expect because great pains are taken to avoid such a disaster. But if falls should occur in such patients, they will often not attempt to walk again, exemplifying Cicero's words:

'Tum pavor sapientiam omnem mihi ex animo expectorat.'
i.e. 'My mind which fear had then oppressed,
Was of all judgement dispossessed.'

THE LAST DROP

Some falls in old people are labelled premonitory falls (Howell, 1971) which precede a sudden and fatal illness, which, however, should not surprise readers who have followed this chapter so far.

MANAGEMENT OF FALLS

As with any disability in old age the essence of successful management is teamwork. On the medical side, the presence of an informed and caring general practitioner, who will see the patient promptly, refer for specialist opinion if necessary and continue to share in the treatment plan, is the keystone of the bridge of care. Many hospital-based specialties may also be required to provide services. The occurrence of falls is frequently the signal for radical changes in the social environment, for example, rehousing, additional home help and other social support, community nursing, physiotherapy, occupational therapy, day hospital treatment etc.

As for my own specialty of geriatric medicine, I can say I think we help, we certainly try. I am indebted to all my colleagues in the specialty without whose painstaking research and thought this chapter would not have been written. In no other branch of medicine does the old aphorism strike so clear a note: 'The greatest clinical challenges are not necessarily presented by rare disease, but by those common illnesses which present in an atypical manner'.

References

Brit. Med. J. (1979). Two geriatric cases. **1,** 1768.
Caird, F. I., Andrews, G. R. and Kennedy, R. D. (1973). Effect of posture on blood pressure in the elderly. *Brit. Heart J.*, **35,** 527.
Finestone, A. J. (1982). *Evaluation and Clinical Management of Dizziness and Vertigo.* (Bristol: John Wright).
Harper, C. (1979). Wernicke's encephalopathy. *J. Neurol. Neurosurg. Psychol.*, **42,** 226–31.

Howell, T. H. (1971). Premonitory falls. *Practitioner*, **206**, 327–30.

Jonas, S., Klein, I. and Dimant, J. (1977). Importance of Holter monitoring in patients with transient cerebral symptoms. *Ann. Neurol.*, **1**, 470–4.

Maclennan, W. J., Hall, M. R. P. and Timothy, J. I. (1980). Postural hypotension in old age. *Age Ageing*, **9**, 25–32.

Overstall, P. W. (1978). Falls in the elderly. In Isaacs, B. (ed.) *Recent Advances in Geriatic Medicine*, p. 65. (Edinburgh: Churchill Livingstone).

Overstall, P. W., Imms, F. J., Exton-Smith, A. N. and Johnson, A. L. (1977). Falls in the elderly related to postural imbalance. *Brit. Med. J.*, **1**, 261–4.

Prudham, D. and Evans, J. G. (1981). Factors associated with falls in the elderly. *Age Ageing*, **10**, 141–6.

Rai, G. S. (1982). Cardiac arrhythmias in the elderly. *Age Ageing*, **11**, 113–15.

Roberts, M. A., Godfrey, J. W. and Caird, F. I. (1982). Epileptic seizures in the elderly. *Age Ageing*, **11**, 24–34.

Szabadi, E. (1984). Neuroleptic malignant syndrome. *Brit. Med. J.*, **288**, 1399.

Sheldon, J. H. (1960). On the natural history of falls in old age. *Brit. Med. J.*, **2**, 1675.

Taylor, I. C. and Stout, R. W. (1983). Is ambulatory electrocardiography a useful investigation in elderly people? *Age Ageing*, **12**, 211–16.

Visser, H. (1983). Gait and balance in senile dementia of Alzheimer's type. *Age Ageing*, **12**, 296–301.

5

Rehabilitation of Fallers

A. SQUIRES and D. E. BAYLISS

INTRODUCTION

Although much has been written on the intrinsic causes of falls little has been documented on the extrinsic factors which generally lead to falls where there is a pre-existing intrinsic factor (Sim, 1984).

Falls can occur at any age and at any time, but there is an increasing incidence with age as reactions become slower, sight and hearing deteriorate, and various pathological conditions progress to cause dizziness and weakness. With increasing age the proportion of falls due to tripping decreases while the proportion due directly to deteriorating health increases (Overstall, 1978). Excluding the pathological conditions which are dealt with fully elsewhere in this book (pp. 15–43, 75–83), much can be done to make the person and the environment safer and lessen the incidence of falls.

Because of the low status afforded by our society to the disabled and elderly the potential faller is unlikely to ask for help in advance. In fact the majority are probably unlikely to seek help even when they have fallen unless they are injured or unable to get up. For this reason we need to enquire sensitively about any falls our patients may have had, even though they may have been referred for other reasons. Falls are often poorly described by the patient and a diagnosis of 'falls' is little help to a therapist who needs to know how, when, where and how often they occur, in the hope that a pattern will emerge. A history of falls may be obtained in 44% of women and 24% of men over the age of 65 living at home (Sim, 1984).

In many cases falls in the home can be prevented by simple 'commonsense' measures. One of the reasons that these measures are seldom undertaken is that most people are creatures of habit and continue to live

45

life in the same patterns in spite of physiological changes with ageing. For example, many older people take great risks in hanging curtains while balancing on a chair and do not ask for help in their wish to maintain standards. It is difficult for families or friends to suggest alternative ways of carrying out tasks without demeaning the person concerned and lowering their self-esteem as an independent person.

PREVENTION

A survey by Issacs (1979) has shown that fallers are more likely to have a further fall, enter hospital and die in the year following the fall, and therefore prevention of falls and of the life-threatening consequences such as hypothermia, pressure sores and pneumonia are essential; 50% of fallers are alone at the time of the fall and two-thirds of accidental deaths in the elderly at home are caused by falls (Gryfe, Amies and Ashley, 1977).

The lack of confidence felt by any of us after a fall is amplified in the elderly who may be seen typically leaning back, gripping the arms of the chair in which they are sitting and showing anxiety by their expression. Any attempts to stand such a person will usually mean that the tightly held chair comes too. Prising him out of a chair will do nothing for his confidence or for the image of the therapist. Confidence in the therapist must first be gained. This may be achieved during exercise sessions where arm, leg and trunk-strengthening exercises are undertaken in the sitting position thus posing no threat to the patient initially.

When the time is right for mobility to commence, many hands should be available as a fall at this stage would be catastrophic. Once the patient gains confidence in his increasing ability and developing independence, further rehabilitation can take place. This lack of confidence must not be underestimated and is often the cause of lost mobility, rather than the fall itself. The gait may also show the backward leaning posture with shuffling steps and the patient may indeed have the classical *timor cadendi* (phobic fear of falling).

Occasionally one comes up against an overconfident patient who will be a falls risk for this reason. Allowing the patient to fall harmlessly may be the shock treatment that is needed to make him safer and prevent a fall at home. This can be done by having two or three experienced staff, all made aware of the routine, available to lower the patient gradually to the floor when he lurches or leans and begins to fall. A few minutes sitting on the floor may make him aware of the risk he is running by his carelessness.

PHYSICAL PREVENTIVE MEASURES

Feet

A glance at the footwear worn by many elderly people can often pinpoint the cause of falls. Women tend to fall more than men and it has been postulated that this could be due to the variety of heel heights and shoe fashion shapes they have worn and the final problem of painful feet (Isaacs, 1979). A recent survey showed that 75% of fallers wore slippers as compared with 4% who wore shoes (Kinsman, 1983). High-heeled shoes reduce the foot contact with the floor, so sensory input is also diminished. Flat, supportive shoes should be encouraged and note taken of worn heels which will also affect balance (Hughes, 1983). Adequate foot support and protection can be provided by some slippers, and indeed they may be the only reasonable answer for painful deformed feet which are little used. Several firms produce shoes in wide fittings, but even these will be of little help unless fitted correctly and the patient able to get them on and off independently. A variety of fastenings are available to replace laces if these cannot be manipulated, and modern shoes may already have velcro fastenings fitted as a fashion trend. Where there is no alternative to a caliper being fitted the patient must be able to get it on and off independently. Suitable fastenings and practice are essential otherwise it will not be worn, and a further hazard is created.

Painful feet will not welcome mobility, and advice from a state-registered chiropodist is essential. Shoes may be discarded for slippers and even abandoned altogether if toenails grow too long for them to be worn.

Leg Length

Unequal leg length can cause poor balance and is easily adjusted. The commonest cause is following hip surgery where the affected leg may become unequal in length. Osteoarthritis of hip and/or knee, rickets, old injuries or congenital deformities may also be seen.

Patients may have adapted to longstanding deformities and a raise may in fact cause a greater hazard. Patients recently undergoing hip surgery should always have their leg length checked and the appropriate shoe raise applied. It may well be that this has been provided in the orthopaedic department to a previously comfortable shoe which now cannot be worn due to postoperative oedema. An excellent immediate solution is the temporary shoe raise which will also test the patient's compliance before an expensive order is executed (Squires and Morris, 1984).

Some patients find a raised shoe aesthetically unacceptable even though orthotists go to considerable trouble to conceal the alteration. It may be helpful to suggest ladies wear trousers to make it less obvious. The patient has, of course, the right to refuse, but mentioning the fact that they will be much more obvious bobbing up and down or lying flat on the floor after a fall may win the day!

To measure leg length the patient is viewed from behind and the examiner places each index finger on the iliac crest. The amount of shortening is measured by placing appropriate size blocks under the foot until the iliac crests are level (Goodwill, 1983).

Walking Aids

Walking aids can be a great help in preventing falls when correctly prescribed and the user taught to use them. Unfortunately many falls are caused because of the walking aid. A great variety of heights, widths and handles are now available, and some may have wheels to assist mobility. Advice should be sought from the rehabilitation department before an aid is purchased and many are available on prescription. Walking sticks, which are more easily and more frequently bought over the counter, cause just as many problems and often resemble shepherds' crooks rather than walking aids. A survey by Sainsbury and Mulley (1982) found that only 22% of sticks assessed had been measured, and of these two-thirds were considered incorrect – the main fault in being too long. Of the patients assessed in the survey who were fallers 75% had sticks of incorrect height which is significant. The handle of the aid should be level with the greater trochanter, but this may be varied by the therapist depending on the patient's condition. Worn ferrules are often the cause of slips and should be replaced with a good quality 'suction' type when showing signs of wear.

If thoughtless prescribing means that an aid will not go through a door the patient will probably discard it or use it incorrectly thus providing another safety hazard.

The patient's gait must be as safe as possible. A feature of the elderly is multiple pathology which means that several problems may be causing poor gait and a compromise may have to be reached. Practice on all types of surfaces should be tried, and movement on stairs and steps should be practised if they are to be encountered at home or in the normal course of day-to-day life.

Unfortunately furniture grabbing and aids do not give correct sensory imput and this should be borne in mind when prescribing aids.

Balance

Balance must be one of the most complex systems in the body, fighting a continual battle against gravity to prevent us from falling. The human body is unstable in the upright position and is only kept there by continuous information from all the sensory receptors. Any fault in any of the systems giving auditory, proprioceptive, visual and touch information will cause the body to be unbalanced. Likewise any fault in the speed of conducting this information will cause imbalance. Impairment in the execution of orders to regain balance, as in neurological conditions or amputation, will prevent balance occurring and a fall may occur. Speed of sway has been found to be greater in fallers than in a comparable group of non-fallers (Fernie *et al.*, 1982). Women also adopt a smaller standing and walking base (Azar and Lawton, 1964).

Balance can be re-educated from sitting to standing to walking using a mirror for visual feedback. It is frequently the most difficult function to re-educate because of its numerous components. But the rewards are well

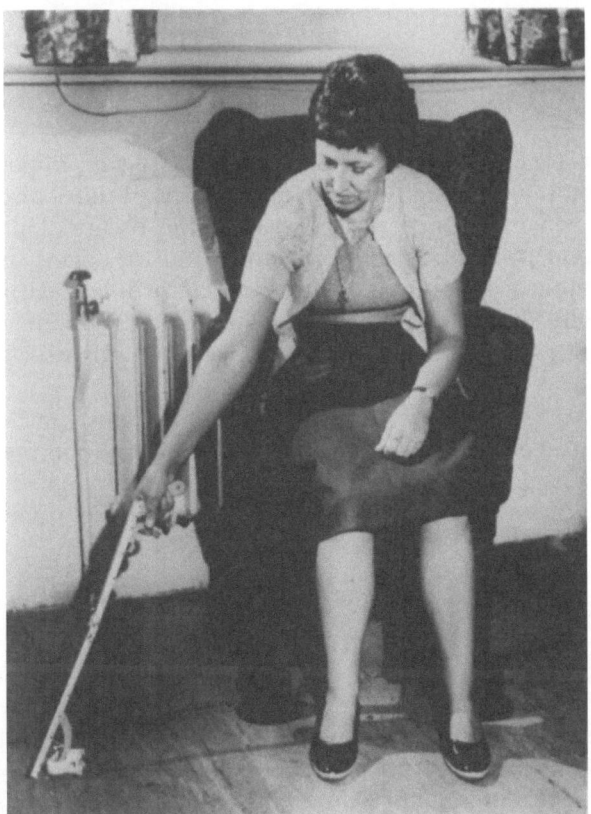

Figure 5.1 'Helping hand'

worth the effort. It must be a team effort with each member aware of what the aim is and why their contribution and vigilance is essential. The relatives must also be drawn in where possible. The correct chair, shoes and walking aid must be available from the start if success is to be possible, and practice with all these items available and named for the patient on the ward with the cooperation of the nursing staff will speed recovery and discharge.

Reaching for objects from the floor can be difficult with disturbed balance; a letter box inside the door will catch the post or a 'helping hand' can pick up small objects (Figure 5.1).

When dressing, reaching forward to put on knickers, stockings or shoes may be difficult. There are a variety of aids for socks or stockings and long-handled shoe horns are easily available to help putting on shoes. The helping hand is useful in putting pants or knickers over the feet when knees or hips are stiff. Surgical collars reduce the proprioceptive impulses of the position of the head on the body and a wearer entering a dark room is more likely to fall.

Visual Measures

In the Kinsman (1983) audit 80% of fallers had visual impairment, and 42% of these could be helped. Glasses may be out of date, dirty or loose – they may not even have been prescribed for the owner! Up-to-date eye checks are a good preventive measure and some opticians may visit the housebound. Bifocals may present a particular problem with steps. The blind and partially sighted will need their hands to feel their way around, and may do better with rails at home than walking aids which will isolate them.

Edges of steps can be clearly marked and light bulbs can be washed or replaced with those of a higher wattage by a supporter. Windows should be clean and curtains allowing as much light in as possible. The stairs in particular should be well lit. Charities for the blind are a good source of help.

Auditory Measures

In the Kinsman (1983) survey 50% of fallers had deafness and 35% could be helped. Poor hearing often goes with poor balance either from the cause of the deafness or because the sufferer worries that the telephone or doorbell have been ringing for some time and rushes to answer them. Hearing checks are available in health districts, and hearing aids do need frequent attention. The deaf owner must have nimble fingers to manipulate the batteries, switches and earpiece. Flashing lights to replace door bells are just one suggestion to aid the deaf, and there are many telephone adaptations available. Charities for the deaf are a good source of help.

Sensory Measures

A person who has suffered a stroke is at particular risk of falling. The constraints to normal mobility caused by spasticity and lack of motor function are obvious and the disturbance of normal righting and equilibrium reactions are a major cause of difficulties in ambulation. These are greatly lessened by early physiotherapy. A graded system of treatment can prevent the patient working beyond the level of their abilities, falling and losing confidence. The effects of a sensory deficit are not as obvious, but can be totally disabling to the person concerned. Disturbances of sensation can take many forms; lack of tactile and proprioceptive sensation or a diminished appreciation of the stimulus give particular problems. If warning sensations from the arm are not appreciated, the arm or hand may be caught in a doorway or the arm of a chair without the owner realizing. Similarly, steps or uneven surfaces may not be appreciated and so cause a fall. Crossing the street when a patient has a hemianopia or does not appreciate his surrounding space are common hazards. In the home this can also cause difficulties with lack of appreciation of obstacles. Retraining patients to compensate intellectually for perceptual problems is extremely difficult. Visual perception can be so distorted so as to cause the patient to close their eyes and try to cope without any vision at all.

The problems of the lower limb amputee who receives no sensation except through the prosthesis are similar. Balance and ambulation are skills that must be practised to prevent the danger of a fall.

In severe cases of poor balance it may be necessary to get the patient mobile again using a self-propelling wheelchair. This is often a last resort for the therapist, the patient and the family because of the inconvenience it causes, but it should be considered and can often allow the patient an independent fall-free lifestyle if the chair is properly prescribed, transfers and wheelchair mobility correctly taught, and any home alterations undertaken in advance.

Muscle Weakness and Joint Stiffness

The arthritic patient also has problems with balance due to muscle weakness and stiff joints and indeed in any patient where a thorough assessment has found these to be lacking a specific treatment programme can be initiated. General and local muscle weakness are common causes of falls (Howell, 1982). Functional exercises are most effective – after all the patient will be living at home, not in a rehabilitation department.

Walking, chair drill, on and off the bed and up and down the stairs will help functionally and specific treatment for particular problems that have been isolated will be necessary. Extended bedrest following a fall leads quickly to muscle weakness and disuse atrophy and should be discouraged unless considered medically essential. Complete bed rest has been found to result in loss of strength of approximately 3% a day or 18–20% a week (Payton and Poland, 1983).

ENVIRONMENTAL HAZARDS

Good design can avoid many of the hazards built into typical housing, including easy access to all rooms, but particularly the bathroom and lavatory. Doorways and passageways should be wide enough for easy access and doors positioned and hung conveniently. Ideally there should be no odd steps or stairs, windows and doors should be easy to manipulate and power points accessible.

The layout of kitchen equipment is important as is storage; other considerations are suitable sanitary equipment, such as WCs and basins, and appropriate floor finishes.

Many of the elderly live in poor accommodation, such as older rented properties with outside lavatories, awkward steps and stairs. The rent may be low and not cover the landlord's cost of repairs. In owner-occupied property there can be problems in organizing repairs or in having the means to fund them. This is a particular problem, for example, for a widow whose husband would have previously done the 'do-it-yourself' jobs in the home. Innovative schemes are being tried to help with these problems. Older people living in council property may also experience difficulty getting necessary repairs done because of the bureaucratic procedures and, possibly, the absence of a telephone to keep contacting the relevant department.

Typical Problems

Entrances to both houses and flats can be hazardous. Cracks and breaks in concrete paths will given an uneven surface which can precipitate a fall. Access to an outside lavatory can be particularly dangerous in wet or icy weather. It is easy enough for anyone to miss their footing on an uneven step. Steps need to be repaired to give an even surface and rails supplied for support where necessary.

Putting out the milk bottles seems to cause a large number of falls and this could be prevented by putting bottles on a shelf or table, or using a long-handled bottle stand so it can be raised or lowered with the bottle in it. The practice of stooping down on icy steps with one foot on the front-door sill, and one on the front door step while hanging onto the door frame should be strongly discouraged. One reason for falling on stairs is that the foot is not completely placed on the stair, and knocking the toe against the riser when ascending and knocking the heel back against the riser when descending will check the position of the climber's feet.

A carpet which is not firmly fixed to the stair creates an additional hazard and such a carpet in a poor state of repair is even worse. An extra bannister rail can be provided to give one on each side, and they should be level and firmly fixed to the wall giving space between rail and wall for the fingers to grip round the rail securely. An extra rail and a simple grab rail placed horizontally on a newel post where there is a turn in the stairs, can make the upstairs of the house more safely accessible. Most social services departments will put up rails if they have the permission of the owner of the property. Rails should extend beyond the step both at the top and at the bottom of the stairs. Systems for doing this and the charges to the client will vary from area to area depending on local policy. This is a major measure in preventing falls.

A stair gate may have its use in preventing known fallers rolling down a flight of stairs, but the dangers of a confused patient trying to climb over it must be considered. If stairs are very dangerous it may be appropriate to put up a physical barrier to block them off completely. Alternative ways of going upstairs and downstairs could be investigated once it has been agreed that using the stairs is a necessity. Overstall (1978) found that three-quarters of falls on the stairs occurred when descending. Methods of going up and down include doing so sideways or in the sitting position, or walking down backwards. A chair may be kept on any landing en route for a rest and a walking aid will be required on each level if normally used. Bringing furniture to one level may be possible and is safer.

Toilet Access

In older property this was sited for convenience of plumbing, not for easy access. The lavatory therefore may be outside, up or down steps or fitted into a corner. Access to the lavatory can be a major hazard for many people. A common fault is that the 'smallest room' has the smallest door, particularly in council and converted flats. In terms of use this is not logical as it is the one room everyone has to use. Widening the doorway can be a difficult and expensive building operation. It may be possible to rehang the door to give better access, or to remove the door and architrave and provide a sliding door or curtain, although neither of these solutions give as much privacy as a door. However, when a lavatory is completely inaccessible a chemical closet, as used when caravanning or camping, may be the answer. These are usually provided by social services departments if not bought privately, but there are problems of safety in their use and difficulties in emptying them if family are not available. Rails in the toilet are always useful and prevent people hanging onto inappropriate items such as the basin, toilet-roll holder or towel rail. Raised seats (Figure 5.2) are helpful for those unable to lower to the traditional height, and the toilet roll and chain should be within easy reach.

Modern lavatory seats tend to be low, designed at this height to aid elimination. However, for many older or disabled people a higher seat is easier to get on and off. The optimum height for the individual can only be judged by assessment but is usually between 46 and 50 cm above floor level. A commercially available raised lavatory seat placed on a lavatory may bring it up to an appropriate height, but there are problems with so

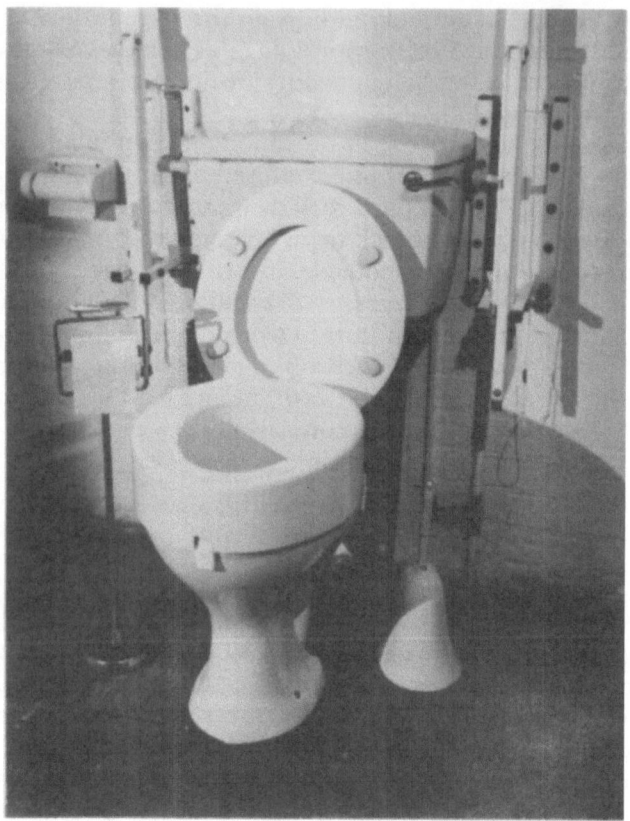

Figure 5.2   Raised toilet seat

much of the seat being above the level of the flush in terms of hygiene. A rail on the wall or walls may give great security and assistance in sitting and standing but the walls must be solid. The recommended height above the floor, sloping down at 30° for a 40 cm rail, is 1100 cm. A quick and easy answer which avoids any fixing to the wall is a Scandia frame; this incorporates a raised seat with its own rails (Figure 5.3). As it is not fixed to the floor care has to be taken in only providing it for people who will be safe pushing up on the middle of the rail to stand, with no danger of tipping the frame. Other safety factors include extending the lavatory chain to within easy reach to avoid overbalancing when looking up; having the toilet roll accessible; having clothing which is easily removed and replaced; and avoiding having an inward-opening door so that if a fall should occur the faller does not inadvertently barricade himself in.

For night-time needs it may be better to avoid going to the lavatory when many factors are present to precipitate a fall, for example, influence of sleeping tablets, poor lighting, hypotension on getting upright from being horizontal in a warm bed, lack of attention to footwear, dangling dressing

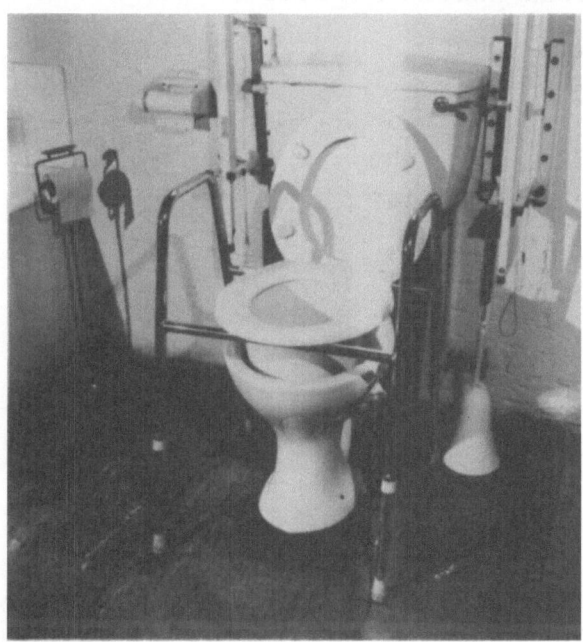

Figure 5.3 Scandia frame

gown cord, etc. Fine (1959) felt that the large number of night falls was due to the need to micturate at night. A suitable commode or urine bottle adjacent to the bed should be considered. Female urinals (Figure 5.4) are not easy for most women to accept or use, but there are a variety available. The do-it-yourself solution of a chamberpot or bucket, or a funnel (or oxygen mask) emptying into a container should be used with care as none will help poor balance. All these solutions are sometimes not easy to accept and must be suggested in a sensitive manner to save embarrassment to both parties.

Falls frequently happen when transferring onto a commode. This is an activity which must be carried out with 100% accuracy every time particularly if the person lives alone. This seems often not to be fully appreciated by hospital staff who may continue to take the patient to the toilet in the night right up to the eve of discharge. As a rough rule of thumb people should transfer out of bed on to the commode towards their strongest side, and back into bed towards their weakest side, so that if they fall towards the weakest side, which is most likely, it will be on to the bed. A one-arm commode which fixes to the bed may overcome this problem and give a safe means of coping with excretion during the night, although the close proximity of the commode may be found offensive. Bedside commodes should either have no wheels, or if present they *must* be locked.

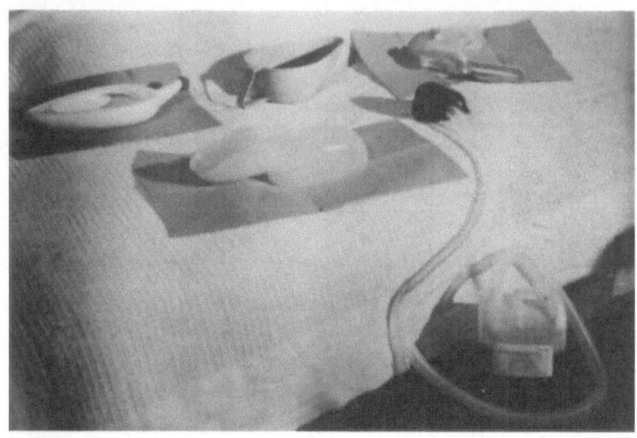

Figure 5.4   Female urinals

A low-watt bulb accessible from the bed by a pull cord may aid safety. A night light constantly on, or neon plug, may be useful, and any risk of dribbling urine en route to the commode must be avoided to prevent a slippery surface forming.

When people are totally unsafe to move around some other means of safe excretion must be considered such as catheterization or long-term sitting on a commode wheelchair so that they can remain at home. For the person whose environment is too hazardous for them the only answer may be a very basic one-room existence.

There are many older people who manage like this; their situation may not be ideal but may be preferred to giving up their home altogether.

Space in a home can be limited. The restrictions of design can be made worse by furniture which is too large or unsuitable for the home. Hallways are often long and narrow in older property and are made even narrower with hallstands, chests or other furniture. This is a particular hazard with wheelchair users when the width of a doorway may be satisfactory but the width of the passage way too small to accommodate the diagonal of a wheelchair (about 1 metre or $3\frac{1}{2}$ ft) which is needed for turning.

Other Hazards

The living room also contains hazards for fallers. Draught excluders should be fastened to the door, not 'sausages' left like a trip wire. Castors on furniture should be avoided as they may move when lent on for support. Although not ideal, many older people are happy to move around their rooms holding onto furniture rather than using a walking aid. If the furniture is solid, this may be accepted and in cramped accommodation there may be little room for an aid. On the whole loose mats are to be avoided but are often deemed to be an essential part of the decor and placed in every doorway. They are aptly named 'slip mats' as in fact they usually do. If the owner cannot be persuaded to remove them, then nailing, sticking or using non-slip matting underneath may help.

Chair drill is a most important procedure for the patient, relatives and care staff to master as it is when approaching the chair that a good many falls occur. The same procedure should be used when getting on and off the toilet. The prerequisites are a suitable chair (height, arms, slant of back and seat), a non-slip floor, adequate strength and joint range, and a reason to move. The chair most likely to be used at home may need adaptations.

Chair Drill and Toilet Drill

The seat should first be the correct height for the patient; the feet should be flat on the floor with the knees at 90°, and should be apart and slightly under the chair, with the hands on the front of the arm rests (Figure 5.5a). The patient wriggles to the front of the chair, then leans forwards and upwards and when upright puts her hands on the walking aid positioned ready in front of her (Figures 5.5b and c). If assistance is needed it should be in the form of encouragement, and helping the patient up and forwards rather than pulling her from in front which is more likely to produce an extension reflex. The subject should allow time for the blood pressure to stabilize before moving, as postural hypotension when moving quickly from sitting (or lying) to standing is a common problem amongst the disabled and also a cause of falls.

When approaching the chair or toilet to sit down the person should not actually sit – until the legs are against the seat, then he or she should put the hands on the arms of the chair, and lower down onto it slowly.

These activities must be practised continually and correctly so that patients by the time they go home carry them out as a matter of habit.

The height and stability of the chair is important and will vary with the requirements of the individual. Dining table chairs, for example, have a height of between 46 cm and 53 cm and are easy to get out of for many people, and the height of the chair should equal the length of the lower leg

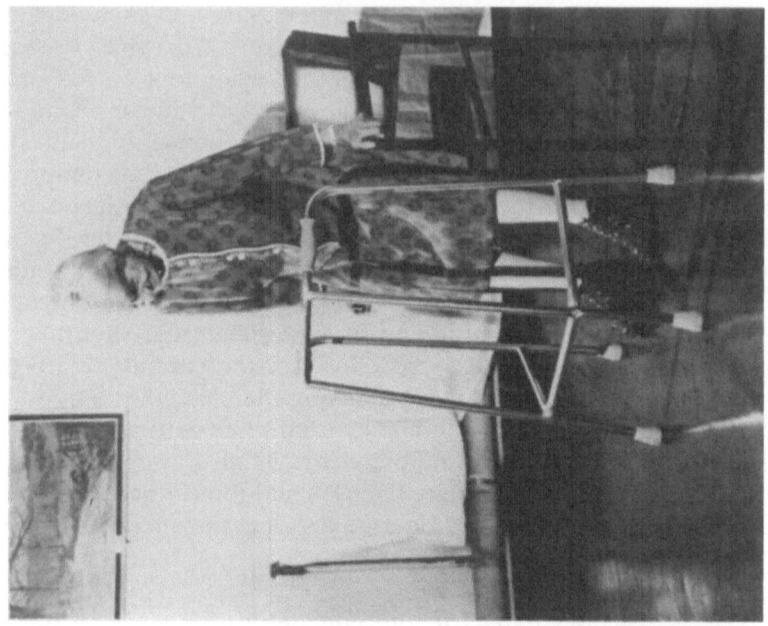

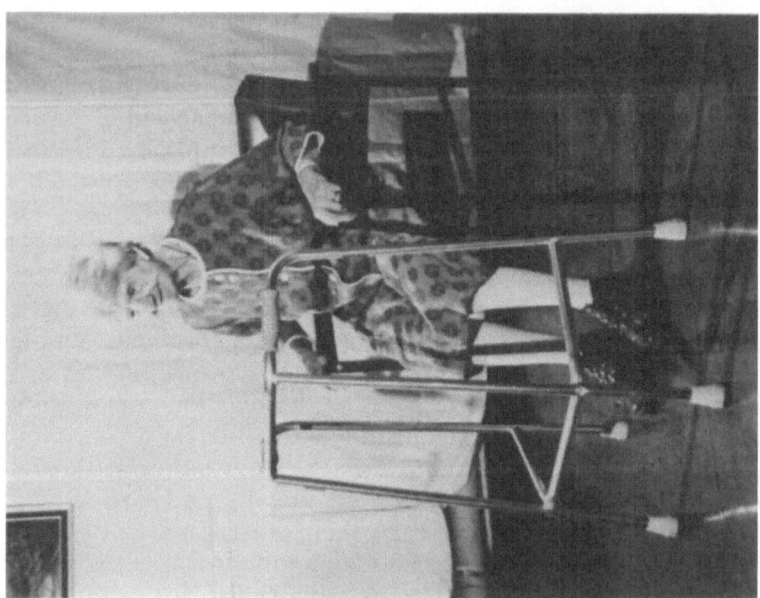

Figure 5.5 (a) and (b)   Chair drill – the correct procedure for raising from a chair

when in the sitting position, with the knee at 90°. Too deep a seat may be comfortable to sit in but can lead to women, in particular, being marooned in the seat and unable to get up due to their comparatively shorter femurs. Chair arms should extend slightly forward for pushing on.

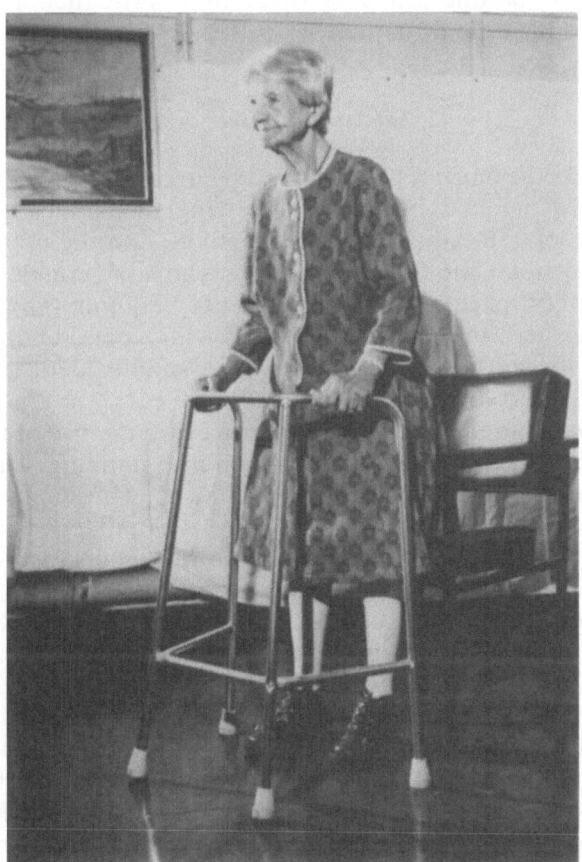

Figure 5.5 (c)

Chairs are expensive items of furniture and not all social services departments will provide them. But often adaptations can be successfully undertaken so that the person's own chair can be retained. These include a wooden board under the cushion to give a firmer 'push off', and a variety of chair raisers are available to fit onto the legs of the chair to attain the correct height. If the family decide to purchase a chair, it must be tried out first, and if the person cannot get out of it unaided in the shop they will be unable to get out of it at home.

If the chair has a tendency to move backwards then it should be placed against a wall for safety. Ejector type seats have met with a mixed response; they can eject the person before his slow reactions have had time to adjust and so cause a fall. The weight of the ejector seat springs are adjustable and may benefit from professional assessment. A 'Kirton' chair for the hypermobile confused person who is also a falls risk incorporates a low backwards slanting seat and these may have their place to restrict mobility with this type of patient.

Safety in the Bedroom

Safety in the bedroom can be improved by organizing the furniture to give easy access to the bed, wardrobe, dressing table, etc. Sometimes it is difficult for people to adjust to getting into bed on the opposite side from their habitual side, but this may be necessary. A double bed, although taking up a lot of space, can often be safer to 'fall' into (and not fall out of) than a smaller bed, but a decision on this will depend on individual needs and choices. It can be hard to adjust to a smaller bed, and the risks of turning over and rolling out are greater.

Standing up from the bed can be improved by the use of fracture boards under the mattress to give a firmer push off into standing. The height is also important and the bed can be raised by blocks. These must be stable and should be joined together for security. Replacement legs can be fitted on to a divan bed to increase the height. If the bed is on castors it should be placed against the wall so that it does not move.

Furniture can be moved to the side of the bed, or rails fitted to prevent falling, but it must be remembered that adding a rail to the side of the bed can increase the height from which the person falls. Confused patients who are likely to fall out of bed frequently could have a mattress laid alongside the bed as a night 'landing pad' to lessen the impact. Rails to assist in standing can be fixed to the bed or to the wall. Health district medical loans departments should be able to provide hospital beds for home use, and innovative schemes in some hospitals are very useful in reclaiming old hospital beds and cutting them down to the exact height needed. All patients should be encouraged to go to bed at night as failure to do this causes lower limb oedema (even on a transatlantic flight without elevation of the legs this can be a problem at any age); often the fear of being incontinent or being unable to get in and out of the bed precludes this activity. Reclining chairs and beds which sit the patient up mechanically can be considered as an alternative.

Keeping Warm

Keeping warm during cold weather is a problem for older people unless they happen to live in property with fitted carpets, double glazing and central heating. Moving to a modern flat with these comforts can transform a person's life and give freedom from a constant battle against the cold. Coping with coal fires is not easy as coal has not only to be carried into the house, but fireplaces cleaned out and made up, all of which involve kneeling on the floor or bending over. Gas or electric fires are easier to use, but whatever is used energy costs for heating a home all day can take a high percentage out of a weekly pension. If someone is in danger of falling a fireguard is essential. Electric bar fires should be checked to ensure that the element cannot be touched. If outlet sockets cannot be raised the patient must be encouraged to sit when switching the socket on. Gas fires should have the switches on the top for easy ignition. Both the Gas and Electric Boards will advise on adaptations. A quarterly account avoids the problems of feeding a meter although many people are happier to control their expenditure by using a meter; it is best if the meter is fixed within easy reach so that climbing on chairs is avoided. Paraffin stoves can be very hazardous and *should not be used by anyone* unless they reach the British Standard which ensures that the flame goes out if the fire tips over.

Keeping Clean

When asking questions about personal hygiene and cleanliness it is best to ask direct questions such as 'how do you keep clean?' rather than ask leading questions in terms of bathing, as often the patient will give the expected answer even though he or she never takes a bath! Bathing is a hazardous activity and not essential to keeping clean, although it is a pleasing activity and a cultural habit. People can be assisted to safe bathing by the use of rails that can be fitted vertically for getting in and out of the bath, or horizontally, or at a slight angle for use with bath seats. Seats can be fitted over the bath or halfway down inside; but they are often an inadequate compromise and to be safe must be fitted very carefully. Non-slip mats or adhesive non-slip treads are invaluable in preventing falls.

The most difficult part of the activity is getting out of the bath, and rails fitted onto the taps do little to assist raising the trunk over the legs. Being marooned in the bath is a terrifying and embarrassing experience, as well as being very cold, and the best answer may be to have assistance from family or from a bathing attendant provided by the health service. Provision of this service is variable around the country and may be provided by the local authority instead. Alternatively a strip wash may be the best and safest answer and this is easier sitting on a perching stool. Showers can be easy and safe but are a fairly new concept and may not be accepted by older people. Whenever any activity involving water is concerned attention must be paid to any spillages so that a wet floor does not contribute towards a fall.

Kitchen Hazards

Wet floors can also be a hazard in the kitchen where the flooring is often linoleum, and a long-handled mop can help with spills. Falls in the kitchen can be very dangerous and lead to serious injury as the rooms are often small, and much of the furniture has sharp edges, is heavy and does not 'give' with the fall. Loose flex, for example, from a portable electric fire

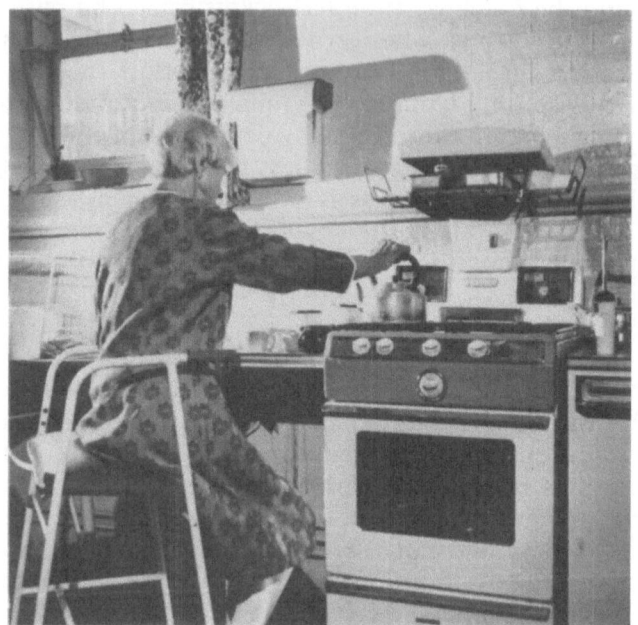

Figure 5.6   Perching stool

can be hazardous. Unsafe use of electric or gas stoves which cause burns may precipitate a fall with the reflex withdrawal response. Leaning down or reaching up into cupboards can cause loss of balance, and storage should be encouraged at levels that are easily accessible. Tea-making equipment is often kept by the hob, as this is easy and efficient. Trays with non-slip surfaces are useful for carrying teacups easily.

Only a small proportion of the total population use their oven (and usually then only on Sundays for the roast), the majority using the top rings. This should be encouraged in the potential faller as reaching down is hazardous. If this activity is agreed to be essential, then sitting on a stool while performing it, or using a raised oven may help. A perching stool is also useful while waiting in the kitchen for food to cook, or stirring or preparing items (Figure 5.6).

It has been suggested that the major problem of older people is moving around the house; the second major problem is carrying things from room to room. A trolley may help with this if it is stable, the right height and has castors which are easy to move but do not roll away too fast and there are no steps en route (Figure 5.7).

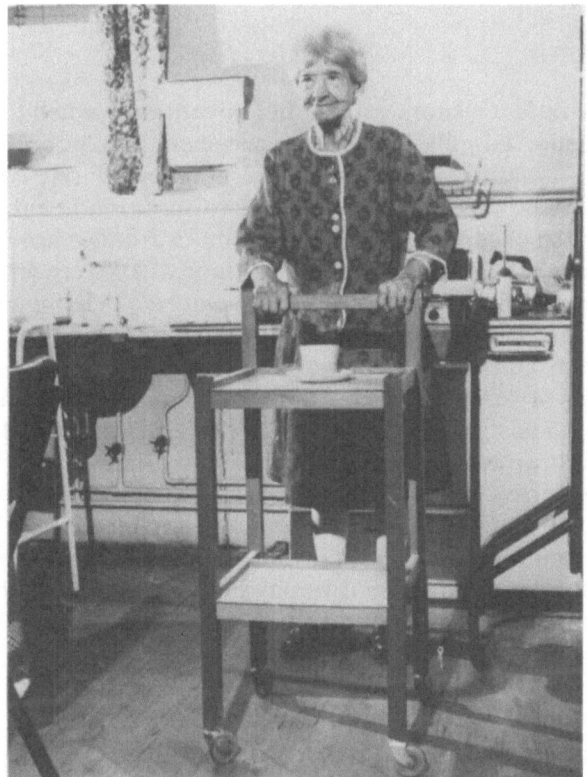

Figure 5.7 Trolley

IF A FALL OCCURS

Even with all the preventive measures outlined a fall may occur for another reason, and the faller and his/her carers will feel more confident if they know how to tackle the problem.

Try to Keep Warm

The secret when you find yourself on the floor after a fall is to keep warm. Pull blankets, coats, rugs and anything else you can find on top of you and under if possible, and either wait for help to come, or consider carefully your next move. Frequent fallers may keep a rug under a chair together with a torch and a bell, which will be much less tiring than summoning help by shouting. A telephone positioned on a low stool, and thus accessible from the floor as well as from a chair, is also a wise precaution.

Try to Get Help

Even those with few visitors will get help eventually when the telltale signs of lights, uncollected milk bottles etc. are seen. The police will be needed to gain access unless keys are held by a neighbour, relative or the social services. It may be possible for the faller to summon help herself by using the phone – if so ensure any relevant numbers are also accessible from the floor. The advent of the cordless phone will overcome the obvious disadvantage of where the telephone is placed. Telephones can be provided under the Chronic Sick and Disabled Persons Act, but are often something that families are willing to provide.

A 999 call will summon help – the emergency services are used to this sort of call for assistance. It does not necessarily mean that the faller will have to go to hospital if the ambulance service comes, but the attendants may feel it is necessary.

A friend or partner in the house may be unable to help the faller and may have to summon help. This may be against the principles of independence inherent in our culture, but it may help to remember that we all have to ask for help at some time and sooner rather than later is always better.

Alarm Systems

There are a variety of specialized aids available but all depend on someone being available to give assistance. In purpose-built accommodation a two-way intercom to a central point may be useful. For the person living alone a small radio transmitter, which can be worn around the neck or in the pocket and can be activated after a fall, may be helpful. This can either automatically ring a series of telephone numbers with a prerecorded message asking for assistance, or be monitored from a control point where someone on duty will ring a series of telephone numbers and if there is no response get someone to visit – maybe the police if no relatives or neighbours are available.

Aids such as this can be invaluable in keeping the 'at risk' person at home for as long as possible. Habit alarms are those which are activated if a common activity is not carried out; this can be not flushing the lavatory for 12 hours or not stepping on to a mat into the kitchen, thus indicating a break in routine needing investigation.

Try to Get Up

Assuming that no apparent injury has been caused by the fall, then there are various methods of getting up which can be tried. Potential fallers referred to rehabilitation departments for treatment could have this included in their treatment programme. The opportunity to practise getting up after a fall before the event occurs is an opportunity we can and should offer to the patient at risk. It is surprising how many enjoy the 'gymnastics' involved. Allowing the elderly and disabled time to do the activity is essential as often they have diminished resources, and it is always useful to remind them that at home they will have as long as they like to get up so there is no rush. If any injury is suspected, moving may be an additional risk and should be restricted; the patient should be kept warm and given nothing by mouth until the doctor arrives.

METHODS OF GETTING UP

Roll and Crawl

The faller needs follow this procedure: roll onto the front, get on to all fours, crawl to a nearby piece of furniture, put the hands on it, bring one foot forward putting the foot flat on the floor, stand up, and sit on the chair carefully to recover (Figures 5.8, 5.9 and 5.10). Crawling, however, is dependent on 'good' knees above almost everything else, and patients with painful knees may be unable to do this. One of the main problems of practising this activity is getting the patient on to the floor to start with and this has been solved by using the Rescue Chair in the reverse mode – that is, sitting on it elevated and lowering it and the patient to the floor, and allowing the patient to wriggle off on to the floor.

Sideways

When crawling is impossible, usually due to painful knees or weakness, the faller may be able to shuffle on the bottom to a piece of furniture, then pull themselves on to the knees and stand up. The knees should be placed centrally in front of the chair to be in the best position.

Using Stairs

When crawling or kneeling are both impossible, shuffling to the stairs, a low stool, suitcase, telephone directory, etc. may be possible, and the faller then gradually moves up and backwards to a height suitable for standing up (Figure 5.11).

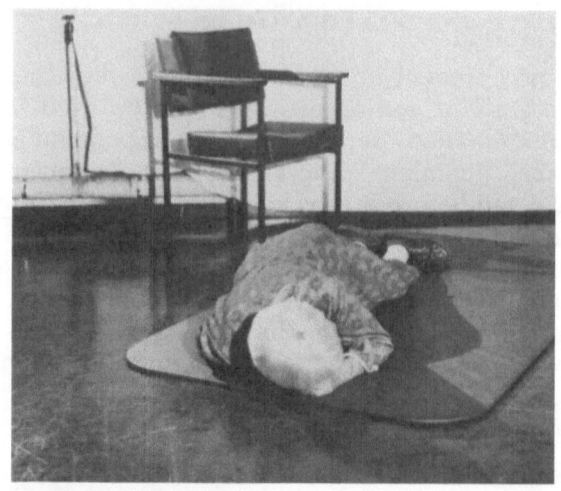

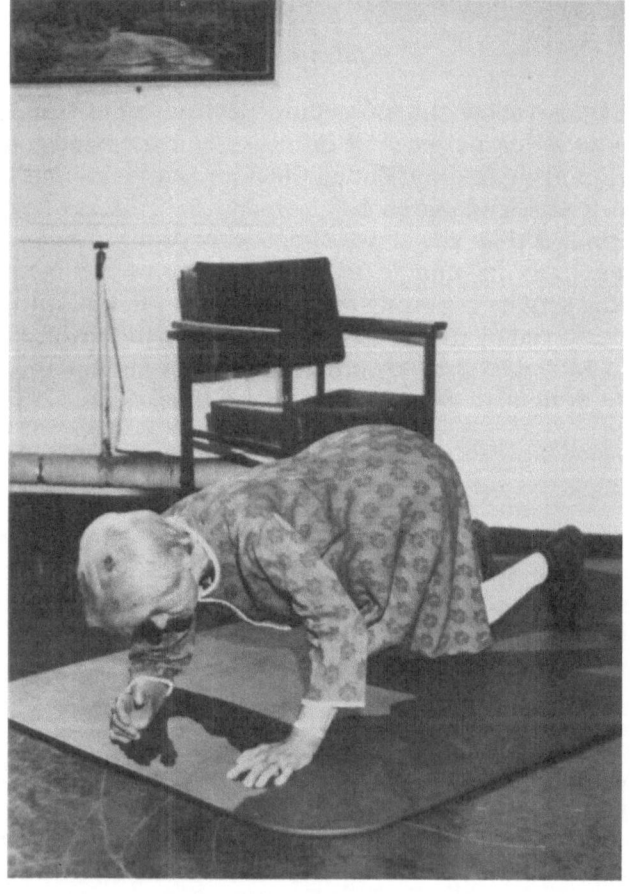

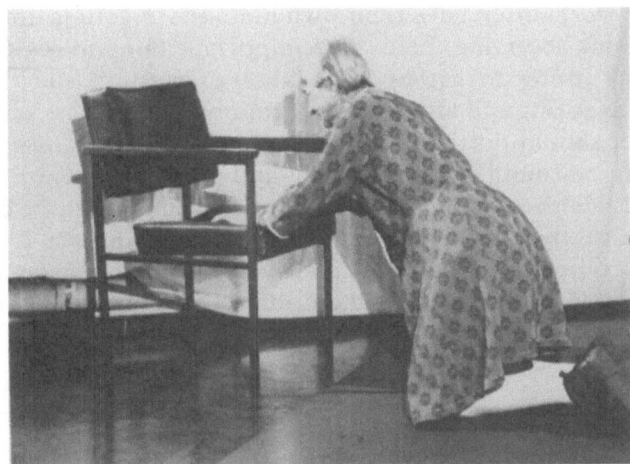

Figures 5.8, 5.9 and 5.10   Methods of getting up – roll and crawl

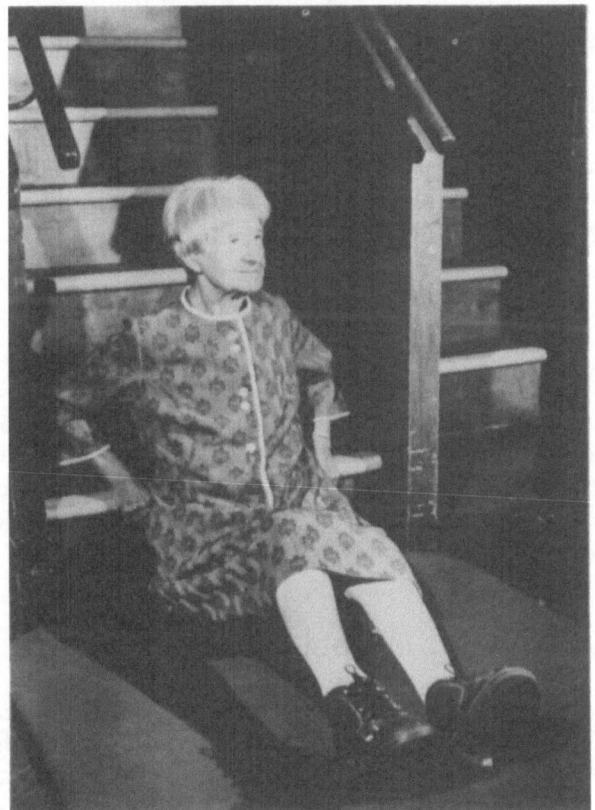

Figure 5.11   Using the stairs to raise to standing

Frequent fallers often have their own methods of getting up and a lot can be learnt from observing them. The important thing to remember is that unsuccessful efforts to get up can cause exhaustion and despondency. Incontinence during and after a fall is common and helpers will accept this, so the faller should not be unduly embarrassed by it. On getting up the faller should rest until she feels ready and safe to move, or she may risk another fall. Helpers needing assistance with lifting should be careful of the method in case they damage themselves. The human body is a very heavy and difficult object to lift, and the emotional tension generated after a fall may mean a greater risk is taken than there would be under other circumstances.

Hoists

Using hoists in the home requires a high level of motivation. Mobile hoists, usually provided by the health service as 'medical loans', are difficult to manoeuvre around the home and take some skill in putting on the slings. Strength is also needed to push the patient and hoist any distance, but it may be the only way of moving someone from bed to chair or chair to commode. They can be used to lift a patient up from the floor but longer chains must be provided for this. Electric hoists are a more expensive item and need to be fitted professionally to the ceiling. These are usually provided by the social services, but again need some skill to be used effectively by a carer.

Rescue Chair

A recent development to help fallers get up from the floor is a chair which is electrically operated by the faller from the floor (Figure 5.12). The seat of the chair is lowered to floor level giving a height of 3″ (8 cm), or ¾″ (2 cm) without the cushion. The faller then wriggles or is helped on to the seat, and presses a switch which takes the seat slowly and quietly up to 21″ (53 cm) from which the majority of patients can stand.

SOLVING PROBLEMS AFTER A FALL

It is much easier to explore the problems caused by falling and try out adapted equipment or different methods of coping when the patient is in hospital, but all suggestions must be relevant to the home situation. In the home it is much harder to implement change. The problems to be considered, although they have similar features, are usually different for each individual as they involve a combination of different factors. These include the person's abilities and disabilities in social, physical and psychological terms, and the advantages and disadvantages of the home situation. The first priority when attempting to solve a patient's problem following a fall is to develop a working relationship in which the patient is treated with respect and their opinions taken account of in an honest and

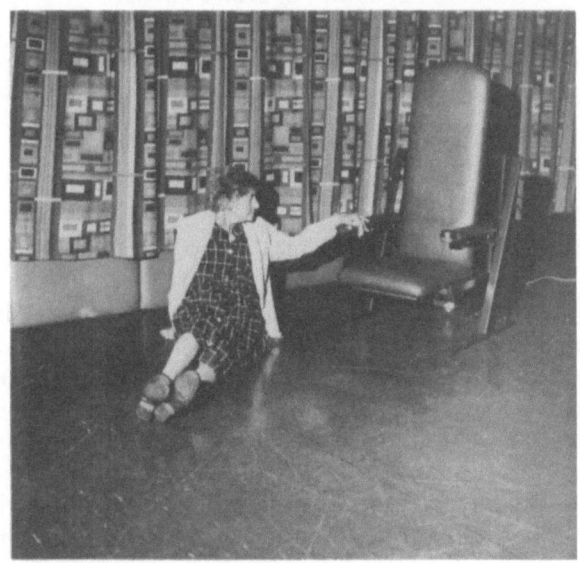

Figure 5.12 Electrically operated 'Rescue Chair'

open way, while still directing them towards joint decisions on future needs. Assessment can only be carried out fully with the patient's cooperation. All members of the team will be able to observe the patient's pattern of movement, and when unsteadiness occurs.

The hospital occupational therapist is uniquely placed to assess the patient in a simulated home environment, as most hospital departments have a small flat or rooms which can represent the average home. They should be adaptable so that rooms can be 'mocked up' to represent the patient's own home as near as possible. This is not always possible, but at least the unit is more like real life than the ward and can be used to gain an initial impression of the patient's abilities. Furniture should be adjustable in height and aids and rails available so that alternative ways of coping can be explored. In addition to observing the patient carrying out everyday activities the therapist should assess physical strength, vision, hearing, coordination and stamina. The length of time during which the patient is seen is important as a patient may perform very well for 5 minutes but become more confused or unstable when carrying out activities over a longer period. This period may be useful to assess perceptual ability and cognitive functions such as concentration, memory, understanding, sequencing of events, etc. in an attempt to discover reasons for falls, or inability to cope, and to seek solutions to the problem.

Activities of Daily Living

Solving problems takes many forms, but when considering many activities of daily living (ADL) it is worth remembering the key words of

avoid
alternative (method)
aid

This is to ensure that other solutions are explored before aids are provided, as a high percentage of aids are never used.

Most people will naturally avoid doing a task which is difficult, but help may be needed to avoid some of the hazards in the home which may not be fully appreciated. They may also not be easy to accept – such as moving to the downstairs of a house, and never being able to go upstairs again. Where falls are likely rails should be provided early on, and not as a last resort; it is better to have a non-essential rail than the danger of a fall.

In broad terms intervention is directed to either improving the patient's functional ability or altering their environment. Functional ability may take the form of treating the patient with exercises and activities to build up confidence, standing balance, range of movements, stamina, power and coordination, or by finding alternative ways of solving the problem. Activities should be carried out in as natural a way as possible. Social activities are highly motivating and should challenge the patient to respond. Altering the environment involves providing aids and adaptations. It is important to remember that many aids are not used, but on the whole safety aids such as rails are well received. If the patient is not involved in the decision-making he or she is less likely to accept the suggested solution.

Overlap within the team to give the patient an integrated and coordinated programme is important and essential in planning for resettlement. There is sometimes some confusion as to whether aids are provided by the NHS or social services departments. A joint aids store can solve this and give an improved service. Provision varies from area to area and some health districts leave voluntary bodies such as the Red Cross to organize this. In broad terms, however, the health service is responsible for providing 'nursing'-type aids such as beds, bed aids, bed rails, cradles, back rests, monkey poles, ripple mattresses, bed-raising blocks and manual hoists, and aids for incontinence such as pads and plastic sheeting. Social services departments are responsible for aids to independence as covered by the Chronic Sick and Disabled Persons Act 1970.

There are often 'grey' areas of 'who provides what' between the two agencies and it is a responsibility, not always treated as a top priority, to ensure that peoples' needs are satisfied, and they are not left in dangerous situations by bureaucracy. Appendix 1 at the end of this chapter shows who supplies what, and when.

PRE-DISCHARGE HOME ASSESSMENT

A more accurate assessment of the patient's ability to cope is seen by taking the patient on a pre-discharge home visit. This may not show a patient's typical pattern of behaviour as it is not a totally real-life situation, and it may well be stressful and provoke anxiety about being 'on trial'. Even so it is likely to give a more accurate sample of the patient's behaviour than that seen in hospital. Patients often behave more naturally in their own home.

Details of the home, such as height of furniture, hazards, etc., can be easily seen. The patient invariably knows where they need rails and during a home visit tailormade solutions can be sought – for example, fitting rails in positions where a patient grabs when falling. More importantly, it is often only on a home visit that problems of concentration, attitudes and low motivation are seen.

The Kinsman (1983) survey found that the average time delay between the most recent falls and referral to physiotherapy was 8.5 days, and two-thirds of these referrals were inpatients. It was also shown that ten to twelve treatments were needed to show a significant improvement, and 64% improved. So early referral and intensive treatment are needed to assist in this problem.

Once the patient is discharged home it is important to consider their continuing care. Increased social support may make all the difference in helping to maintain independence. If having a fall has caused loss of confidence, a volunteer or a 'dial-a-ride' service may be needed for help in going out again.

References

Azar, G. J. and Lawton, A. H. (1964). Gait and stepping as factors in the frequent falls of elderly women. *Gerontologia*, **4**, 83–4.

Fernie, G. R., Gryfe, C. I., Holliday, P. J. and Llewellyn, A. (1982). The relationship of postural sway in standing to the incidence of falls in geriatric subjects. *Age and Ageing*, **11**, 11.

Fine, W. (1959). An analysis of 277 falls in hospital. *Gerontol. Clin.*, **1**, 292.

Goodwill, J. (1983). Low back pain. In Berry, H., Hamilton, E. and Goodwill, J. (eds.) *Rheumatology and Rehabilitation*. (London: Croom Helm).

Gryfe, C. I., Amies, A. and Ashley, M. J. (1977). A longitudinal study of falls in an elderly population. *Age Ageing*, **6**, 201.

Howell, T. H. (1982). Old folks' falls. *Geriatr. Med.*, **12** (11), 61–3.

Hughes, J. (1983). *Footwear and Footcare for Adults*. (London: Disabled Living Foundation).

Isaacs, B. (1979). Fallen women. *Concord*, **14**, 15–23.

Kinsman, R. (1983) *Falls in the Elderly*. Unpublished audit. (London: Barnet Health Authority).

Overstall, P. W. (1978). Falls in the elderly – epidemiology, aetiology and management. In Isaacs, B. (ed.) *Recent Advances in Geriatric Medicine*. (Edinburgh: Churchill Livingstone).

Payton, O. D. and Poland, J. L. (1983). Ageing process. *Phys. Ther.*, **63**, 41–8.

Sainsbury, R. and Mulley, G. (1982). Walking sticks used by the elderly. *Br. Med. J.*, **284**, 1751

Sim, J. (1984). Problems of instability in old age. *J. R. Soc. Health*, **104** (4), 144–6.

Squires, A. and Morriss, M. (1984). Temporary shoe raise. *Physiotherapy*, **70**, 466.

APPENDIX 1: GUIDE TO THE AVAILABILITY OF AIDS AND APPLIANCES FOR PATIENTS CARED FOR AT HOME BY THEIR GENERAL PRACTITIONERS

The provision of aids is often the final solution to a situation in which the patient's condition and ability to cope at home have been assessed. A team approach is helpful, with the patient's relatives, district nurse, physiotherapist, occupational therapist, and health visitor able to contribute constructive suggestions.

Patients Nursed at Home

Beds, bed aids and accessories (mattresses, ripple/polyfloat) — District health authority / Community supplies department

Backrests
Bed blocks, rails, cradles
Bedpans — or
Urinals (male and female)
Transfer boards — Request through district nurse
'Monkey-pole' hoists — Delivery 1–2 days; on loan
Manual hoists

NOTE Request *assembled* bed and mattress (otherwise DIY kit arrives)

Bedpans — British Red Cross Society
Urinals
Feeding cups — Equipment on loan; deposit needed
Air-ring

Patients with Incontinence or Difficult Toileting

Inco-pads   Community supplies department
Inco-pants (plastic or fabric)
Plastic sheeting
Catheters
Commodes (it is essential to check
  who will empty these)

Patients with Mobility Problems

Walking sticks   Community physiotherapist
Elbow crutches
Tripod sticks
Zimmer frames

Wheelchairs ⟨ Temporary   Red Cross

             Permanent   Wheelchair appliance centre (form
                      AOF5G available from DHSS)
                    Rehabilitation officer or adviser
                      (OT) to assess and arrange
                      provision

Aids for Independence

Functional problems can be assessed and solutions explored with the patient. These may involve retraining patients in alternative methods, home adaptations, or provision of aids. It is easiest for the occupational therapist to start with a statement of the problem because sometimes the most obvious solution may not be the most appropriate.

Problems in:
Toileting   Community occupational therapist
Eating   Telephone *social services duty officer*
Kitchen activities   or *area office* stating problem and
Self-care   degree of urgency; delivery time
Bathing   varies but problems with toileting and
Dressing   eating are treated as top priority

    Alterations can be made to property, such as widening doorways, ramping stairs; where the property is unsuitable it can be altered, or rehousing to more suitable accommodation considered.

Musculoskeletal Problems

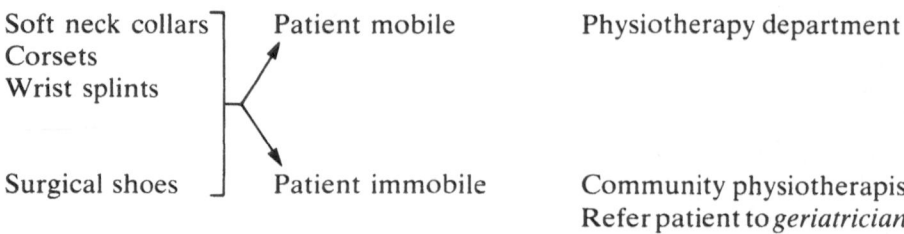

Soft neck collars ⎤   Patient mobile   Physiotherapy department
Corsets
Wrist splints

Surgical shoes   ⎦   Patient immobile   Community physiotherapists
                                                  Refer patient to *geriatrician*,
                                                  or *orthopaedic surgeon*,
                                                  or *rheumatologist*, who
                                                  will arrange for fitting if
                                                  appropriate.

An information sheet for general practitioners devised by Dr Helen Graham, Miss D. Bayliss, BAOT, and Miss B. Davis, MCSP, for King's College Hospital Medical School, Department of General Practice Studies.

APPENDIX 2: USEFUL ADDRESSES

Cosyfeet Slippers, 6 Withey Close, East, Westbury on Trym, Bristol BS9 3SZ (Tel. 0272 681503).

Kirton Chairs, Bungay Road, Hempnall, Norwich, Norfolk, NR15 2NG (Tel. 050842 8145).

Carters (J. and A.) (Walking aids and ferrules), Alfred Street, Westbury, Wiltshire BA13 3DZ (Tel. 0373 822203).

Rescue Chair, Rehab. Products Ltd., Bridge Works, Hasketon, Woodbridge, Suffolk HP13 6HP (Tel. 0473 35475).

Royal Society for the Prevention of Accidents, Priory Queensway, Birmingham (Head Office, Cannon House) (Tel. 021 233 2461).

Ellis, Son and Paramore, (Perching stool), Spring Street Works, Sheffield S3 8PB.

A. W. Gregory and Co. Ltd., Glynde House Street, London SE4 1RY.

Homecraft Supplies, (Aids), 27 Trinity Road, London SW17 7SF.

Masterpiece Products Ltd., (Bed rails), Booth Hill Works, Booth Hill Lane, Oldham, Lancs OL1 2PH

Nottingham Medical Equipment Co., (Aids), 17 Ludlow Hill Road, Melton Road, West Bridgford, Nottingham NG2 6HD.

Renray Products, (Aids), King Street, Cheshire CW10 9LG.

Safe Tie, 15 Meadow Close, High Wycombe, Bucks HP11 RG.

Searle Medical, PO Box 88, Lane End Road, High Wycombe, Bucks HP12 4HL.

J. Spencer and Co. Ltd., (Aids), Moor Road Works, Leeds LS6 4BH.

SML Bath Place, (Aids), High Street, Barnet, Herts EN5 5XE.

Disabled Living Foundation, 380/384 Harrow Road, London W9 2HU (Tel. 289-6111). Display of Aids and Information.

6

Gait and Falls

M. S. KATARIA and S. K. DAS

TYPES OF GAIT

Normal Gait

Normal gait is the manifestation of movement of the human body along a straight line. To perform this, it requires adequate ranges of movement in the joints of the lower limbs (toes, ankles, knee and hip joints), normal muscle power, in extension and flexion of leg muscles, together with high levels of integrated function of the sensory and motor components of the central nervous system.

Abnormal Gait and its Analysis

When a person fails to walk straight in an erect position due to defects in any joints of the lower limbs or lack of postural reflexes in the limbs, and/or in the presence of inadequate muscle power, it results in an abnormal gait.

The following methods are used for research purposes in identification of abnormal gaits and their clinical diagnosis, for example:

Biomechanical Analysis

This is obtained by slow or rapid step by step ciné film movement.

Time and Distance Factors Analysis

This is used for studying locomotion in patients, especially when someone is suffering from joint and locomotor system disease. In disease of joints the velocity of walking will vary, and therefore the length of stride will be affected.

Electromyography

Electromyography and analysis of the muscle fatigue time also reveals various muscle disorders associated with gait abnormality.

In the absence of such sophisticated monitoring facilities, a simple functional assessment is carried out. It is essential that all patients are asked to perform some simple tasks:

1. Rise and transfer from bed to chair, chair to commode, and back to bed again.
2. Rise from chair and walk in a straight line, inside or outside the parallel bar, to return to the point of start, stop in between.
3. Pick up objects from the floor while standing or sitting in a chair.

DISTURBANCES OF EQUILIBRIUM AND GAIT

Dizziness

The patient may complain of recurrent dizziness, sense of rotation and falls. This may be due to a lesion in the internal auditory meatus and semicircular canals.

In cases where the patient fails to walk steadily, and in particular is unable to come down stairs, then the lesion is probably in the labyrinth, in the internal auditory meatus. Such patients also complain of dizzy spells on walking. There is ataxia, but the postural reflexes remain intact.

Ataxia

Due to Loss of Sensation, Limb Weakness, or Cerebellar Disease

Conditions where ataxia may occur due to the above include hereditary, spinocerebellar artery thrombosis, cerebellar degeneration and infarction.

Drug intoxication with sedatives, antiepileptic drugs and alcohol may also cause reversible ataxia. Disease of the cerebellum or its connections may result in difficulty in standing with or without the eyes closed; there is intention tremor and nystagmus. The patient's gait is widespread in disarray like a drunk and he cannot walk in a straight line. When the pyramidal tracts and cerebellar pathways are involved, as in multiple sclerosis, the gait is spastic with ataxia. Very pronounced ataxic gait occurs in the hereditary familial condition of Friedreich's ataxia. The posterior column and spinocerebellar tracts are involved.

Due to Posterior Column Degeneration

This may occur in tabes dorsalis resulting in loss of reflexes, vibration sense, deep pain and a positive Romberg sign. The patient may complain of lightning pains and have Argyll–Robertson pupils. The gait is usually high-stepping and ataxic.

Due to Peripheral Neuritis

When due to peripheral neuritis (motor and sensory involvement) the gait results in slapping of the feet while walking due to foot drop. If only the legs are affected then a walking aid can take the patient's weight. The patient needs to practise control of the ataxic movement and control of foot placement.

Spastic Gait

In upper motor neurone hemiplegia or paraplegia the following conditions can be present.

1. Cerebral infarction or embolism
2. Brain stem lesion
3. Cervical spondylosis
4. Spinal cord compression
5. Parasagittal meningioma, etc.

There is spasticity with weakness, increased reflexes, and usually a positive Babinsky's sign. There is also extensor spasm of the lower limbs with plantar flexion of the foot, and this combined with adductor spasm may cause a crossed or scissor gait.

The steps are short and narrow-based. The upper limb is held in flexion at the elbow and wrist and the spastic limb is externally circumducted to clear the plantar flexed foot and toe off the ground. Prior to gait retraining, spasticity should be reduced if possible by drugs or physical methods, and balance retraining given.

If the condition is longstanding, attempts to improve it may be futile, and making mobility as safe as possible will be the aim. If the condition is new then consideration must be given as in all cases to the realistic aims of treatment, bearing in mind the accommodation and family background, and motivation of the patient.

Marche à Petit Pas

Marche à petit pas (walking with small steps), Petren's gait and apraxic gait may be three stages in a continuum, and the causative diseases for all these are probably similar. 'Marche à petit pas' may follow generalized cerebral arteriosclerosis or multi-infarction of the brain stem, and results in a shuffling gait. There may be accompanying rigidity giving the appearance of a Parkinsonian gait and syndrome. There are many different pathological causes of this typical gait, notably Alzheimer's disease, multi-infarct dementia and normal-pressure hydrocephalus. It should be clearly distinguished from Parkinson's disease.

Petren's Gait or 'Stammering Gait'

This is a variant of the 'petit pas', where a patient with a shuffle gets stuck from time to time and one of the feet does not lift or move forward.

Apraxic Gait

Patients with diffuse cerebral disease may develop apraxia of the lower limbs. There is no loss of power in the limbs and while lying in bed the patient may readily move the legs, but on standing up and attempting to move, the patient cannot carry out walking movements. He does a quick mark time motion without getting anywhere. This has also been called the 'slipping clutch syndrome'. It has been suggested that the parietal lobe may be involved.

The patient's negative and counter reactions to requests to relax a limb are evident. When the examiner tries to flex the knee, the patient extends it and offers resistance (*Gegenhalten*).

Treatment is difficult as the patient is probably unaware of the problem and is not motivated to move. Continued encouragement to stand and walk between two people may at least prevent immobility in bed and thus prevent contractures – leading to a fetal position and a difficult nursing problem.

Frontal Lobe Disorder and Gait

In diseases of the frontal lobe, such as cerebrovascular dementia, Alzheimer's disease and pseudobulbar palsy, patients usually present with a posture of slight flexion, and feet placed further apart than normal. They walk hesitantly and need repeated prompting to continue moving. There is grasp reflex of the hands, while a similar reflex of the feet interferes with walking.

Festinating and Shuffling Gait

This is seen in Parkinsonism, mainly due to dopamine deficiency or a lesion in the extrapyramidal area which may be caused by encephalitis, phenothiazine toxicity, heavy metal poisoning and the punchdrunk syndrome of boxers.

The main disorder of gait in Parkinsonism is rigidity associated with an attitude of universal flexion, such as flexion at the knee and ankle, with flexion at the elbow joints, the small joints of the fingers and pillrolling movements in them. Cerebrovascular disease may simulate the parkinsonian-like rigidity and forward flexion, which stops the patient walking with 'heel first'; he is thus forced to walk on his toes with quick short sloppy dragging steps resulting in recurrent trip-falls.

Dystonia: Athetotic and Choreic Gait

In athetosis, patients often show slow, sinuous writhing movements of the upper limbs, and plantar flexion at the ankles causing maximum weight-bearing on the toes.

At times the patient may present with one arm held aloft, and the other behind the body with slow sinuous movements of the fingers. The head shows titubation, due to extrapyramidal motor disorder.

In chorea, especially Sydenham's chorea, the patient often has a bizarre gait – when trying to advance there is a continuous play of irregular grimacing movement of the face and choreic movement of the neck and hands.

Hemiballismus

This is an example of hemichorea, and affects one side of the body with the leg and arm thrashing about, interfering with walking. The lesion is in the subthalamic nucleus.

Tardive Dyskinesia

This is an example of chorea mainly involving the face and tongue, and it appears as grimacing and tongue-chewing. The chorea may also affect the body. These movements may occur due to some antiparkinsonian drugs and phenothiazines, the effects being dose-related. Neuroleptics, as used in some mental disorders such as schizophrenia, may sometimes cause these movements as an irreversible side-effect.

Muscle Weakness and Myopathic Gait

Weakness of muscles may arise due to muscle disease or disorder secondary to systemic disease, such as osteomalacia, thyrotoxicosis, diabetes, myasthenia, carcinoma and polymyositis. The weakness of the pelvic girdle muscles causes difficulty in walking and climbing stairs. Hypokalaemia due to overzealous diuretic therapy may cause generalized weakness and tendency to fall.

Waddling Gait

This is usually associated with bilateral dislocation of the hips due to congenital familial or genetic-determined disease of muscle and bone. Here the patient has a 'rhumba walk' with alternate dipping of the hip, also resembling a duck or penguin waddle. This kind of gait also occurs with proximal myopathy due to various causes, such as hypokalaemia, diabetes, etc.

Bizarre or Highly Abnormal Gait

This gait does not conform to any normal or recognized pattern. The reaction of the patient is unpredictable. Although a wide variety of bizarre gaits are encountered they are rarely if ever due entirely to a non-organic cause.

TYPES AND RESULTS OF FALL

Forward Fall

A forward fall on the face or shoulder joint may occur when walking with a limping gait and a walking frame. This is usually seen in hemiplegia, or Parkinson's disease, and may result in a fractured nose, fractured surgical neck of humerus, shoulder dislocation or fractured clavicle; rarely, a jaw bone may fracture.

Backward Fall

A backward fall on the occiput may occur in Parkinson's disease and cervical spondylosis, where fracture of occiput or cervical vertebrae may occur.

Fall on Outstretched Hand

A fall on an outstretched hand due to a slip or trip as in Parkinson's disease, impaired eyesight, dark corner, or a slippery mat may occur because of an impaired stagger reflex. A Colles' fracture or fractured clavicle may result.

Crushing Fall

A crushing fall on the buttock or pelvis, usually due to a slip-fall associated with abnormal posture and walking frame fall may cause crush fracture of vertebrae. In fracture of pubic rami, signs like blood per urethra, perineal haematoma, and distended bladder are important to observe.

Fall from a Height

A fall from a height, usually a hospital bed and through or over a cot side, stumbling or missing a step at home or a slip-fall over a loose mattress at home, or shop floor may cause the fractured neck of femur commonly seen in the elderly. In dislocation of hip and unimpacted fracture of the femoral neck the patient cannot stand up, but with an impacted fracture he may walk unaided until a slight trauma causes disimpaction.

MEDICOLEGAL ASPECT OF FAINTS AND FALLS AND CONFUSIONAL STATE IN THE ELDERLY

Falls Outside Hospital

In the case of falls of the elderly disabled people at home or anywhere in the community, it is the domain of the general practitioner to settle issues regarding any injury, and such cases should be referred to the nearest accident and emergency unit for further investigation and assessment. However, many accidents may be reported on a 999 call either to the police or ambulance station.

In the event of a fall contributing to a fatal outcome, the coroner should be notified to determine the cause of death.

In the hospital all falls, however trivial, should be investigated, and in cases of suspected head injury or fracture of long bones, proper investigation and treatment should be given as necessary, and advice from orthopaedic surgeons taken.

Postoperative Trauma Cases

Following trauma, all postoperative cases dying within 1 year are usually reported to the coroner.

Mentally Confused Patients

Death of a mentally confused patient following a fall in hospital should be reported and discussed as necessary with the coroner's department.

Death certificates and cremation papers should be signed by doctors fully registered with the General Medical Council whenever possible, and in the case of cremation papers form 'C' must be signed by a medical practitioner fully registered with the General Medical Council for at least 5 years in accordance with Cremation Acts 1902 and 1982 (England and Wales).

Bibliography and Further Reading

Ashton, F. and Hall, M. R. P. (1974). Cardiovascular diseases in the elderly. *Medicine*, **25**, 1480.

Backett, E. M. (1965). *Domestic Accidents*. (Geneva: World Health Organization).

Bowditch, H. P. (1871). Uber die Eigenthumlichkeiten der reizbarkeit, welche die Muskelfasern des Herzens Zeigen. *Ber. Konig. Sachs. Gesell. Wissenschaften*, **23**, 652.

Brocklehurst, J. C. (1975). Two centre surveys into the cause of fractured femur and its relationship to bone disease. 2. Relevant clinical factors. British Geriatric Society. (Autumn Meeting).

Castle, O. M. (1950). Accidents in the house. *Lancet*, **1**, 315.

Chao, E. Y., Laughman, R. K., Schneider, E. and Stauffer, R. N. (1983). Normative data of knee joint motion and ground reaction forces in adult level walking. *J. Biomech.*, **16**(3), 219–33.

Clarke-Williams, M. J. (1969). The elderly double amputee. *Geront. Clin. (Basel)*, **11**, 183.

Cox, J. R., Adham, A. K., Agarwal, M. L. *et al.* (1973). Postural hypotension: body fluid compartment and electrolytes. *Age Ageing*, **2**, 112.

Doane, N. E. and Holt, L. E. (1983). A comparison of the SACH and single axis foot in the gait of unilateral below-knee amputees. *Prosthet. Orthot. Int.*, **7**(1), 33–6.

Fisher, C. M. (1982). Hydrocephalus as a cause of disturbances of gait in the elderly. *Neurology (NY)*, **32**(12), 1358–63.

Fogel G. R., Katoh, Y., Rand, J. A. and Chao, E. Y. (1982). Talonavicular arthrodesis for isolated arthrosis: 9.5-year results and gait analysis. *Foot Ankle*, **3**(2), 105–13.

Gifford, G. and Hughes, J. (1983). A gait analysis system in clinical practice. *J. Biomed. Eng.*, **5**(4), 297–301.

Jansen, E. C., Vittas, D., Hellberg, S. and Hansen, J. (1982). Normal gait of young and old men and women. Ground reaction force measurement on a treadmill. *Acta Orthoped. Scand.*, **53**(2), 193–6.

Johnson, R. H., Smith, A. C. *et al.* (1965). Effect of posture on blood pressure in the elderly. *Lancet*, **1**, 731.

Judge, T. G. (1968). Hypokalaemia in the elderly. *Geront. Clin (Basel)*, **10**, 102.

Kolstad, K., Wigren, A. and Oberg, K. (1982). Gait analysis with an angle diagram technique: application in healthy persons and in studies of Marmor knee arthroplasties. *Acta Orthoped. Scand.*, **53**(5), 733–43.

Lehmann, J. F., Esselman, P. C., Ko, M. J. Smith, J. C., deLateur, B. J. and Dralle, A. J. (1983). Plastic ankle-foot orthoses: evaluation of function. *Arch. Phys. Med. Rehabil.*, **64**(9), 402–7.

Livesley, B. and Atkinson, L. (1974). Repeated falls in the elderly. *Mod. Geriatr.*, **4**(11), 458.

Minford, A. M., Minns, R. A. and Brown, J. K. (1983). Asymmetry of gait in normal children demonstrated by polarized light goniometry. *Chld. Care. Hlth. Dev.*, **9**(2), 97–108.

Mizrahi, J. Susak, Z., Heller, L. and Najenson, T. (1982a). Objective expression of gait improvement of hemiplegics during rehabilitation by time-distance parameters of the stride. *Med. Biol. Eng. Comput.*, **20**(5), 628–34.

Mizrahi, J., Susak, Z., Heller, L. and Najenson, T. (1982b). Variation of time–distance parameters of the stride as related to clinical gait improvement in hemiplegics. *Scand. J. Rehabil. Med.*, **14**(3), 133–40.

Miyazaki, M., Kitahara, Y., Yorifuji, S., Miki, H. and Fujita, M. (1982). Characteristics of gait ataxia in spinocerebellar degeneration assessed by means of simple quantitative method. *Fol. Psychiatr. Neurol. Jpn.* **36**(4), 401–8.

Murphy, J. and Isaacs, B. (1982). The post-fall syndrome. A study of 36 elderly patients. *Gerontology*, **28**(4), 265–70.

Nayak, U. S. and Gabell, A. (1983). Foot-placement analysis in the elderly – practical considerations. *J. Biomed. Eng.*, **5**(1), 69–72.

Patel, K. P. (1976). Falls and faints in the elderly. *Mod. Geriatr.*, **6**(3), 28.

Pritchard, B. N. C. (1973). Hypotensive agents. *Br. J. Hosp. Med.*, **10**, 45.

Rodstein, M. and Camus, A. S. (1973). Interrelation of heart diseases and accidents. *Geriatrics*, **28**(2) 87–96.

Rosenberg, A. G. (1982). Gait abnormalities following surface hip replacement: a comparative study of patients with surface and total hip replacements. *Proc. Inst. Med. Chic.*, **35**(3), 77–82.

Sheldon, J. H. (1960). On the natural history of falls in old age. *Br. Med. J.*, **2**, 1685–90.

Simon, S. R., Trieshmann, H. W., Burdett, R. G., Ewald, F. C. and Sledge, C. B. (1983). Quantitative gait analysis after total knee arthroplasty for monoarticular degenerative arthritis. *J. Bone Joint Surg. (Am).*, **65**(5), 605–13.

Stillwell, A. and Menelaus, M. B. (1983). Walking ability in mature patients with spina bifida. *J. Pediatr. Orthoped.*, **3**(2), 184–90.

Sudarsky, L. and Ronthal, M. (1983). Gait disorders among elderly patients. A survey study of 50 patients. *Arch. Neurol.*, **40**(12), 740–3.

Wilder, P. A. and Sykes, J. (1982). Using an isokinetic exercise machine to improve the gait pattern in a hemiplegic patient. A case report. *Phys. Ther.*, **62**(9), 1291–5.

7

Community and Hospital Services

M. GREEN

INTRODUCTION

Fits, faints, falls and funny turns (also often largely grouped under the heading of instability), are amongst the giants of geriatric medicine. Along with immobility, incontinence and mental confusion they account for a great proportion of disability affecting older people, and therefore make substantial demands on health professionals and other carers.

Reviewing impact of fits and falls on the general practitioner and primary care team, the community generally (relatives and friends, and statutory and voluntary services) and hospitals, and the interfaces and interplay between and the response of the diagnostic, management/treatment and supportive groups is in effect an overview of the whole of geriatric medicine in and out of hospital. Acute and chronic or acute-on-chronic problems may result from or be caused by these one-off or repeated episodes. They may come into the medical, surgical or psychological domain of doctors, nurses and therapists. The impact of national, local, social and financial policies are important, influencing both their causation and treatment. An effective response to the fit, faint or fall in terms of diagnosis and treatment will depend on general practitioner, ambulance service, and an adequate provision of other appropriate resources. These are, for example, an accident and emergency department geared to the 'clients' likely to present to it, orthopaedic and geriatric bed provision and assessment and treatment and supportive aftercare facilities in the community.

CASE HISTORY

Mrs Smith is a widow, aged 85. She suffers from Parkinson's disease, osteoarthritis and poor eyesight. She often stumbles and sometimes falls both in and out of her house. She has been to the casualty department several times. Luckily she has not hurt herself much, apart from breaking two ribs on one occasion and suffering severe bruising on another. Her daughter is aged 60 and lives in a small flat some miles away. Her general practitioner, social worker and neighbours are concerned that she might suffer a more serious fracture, head injury or be found by the home help lying on the floor dead from hypothermia. Mrs Smith is reluctant to leave her home although it is an old house full of obstacles, and has steps down to an outside toilet.

Response

1. The general practitioner, or practice nurse or geriatric health visitor or a relative should to try and check that the antiparkinsonian drugs are not causing postural hypotension or arrhythmias, or that the drugs for Parkinson's disease and arthritis are not causing confusion.
2. Consider requesting a domiciliary visit by geriatrician and occupational therapist to review medical condition and functional mobility in the patient's own environment. This is often worth doing even when day hospital referral is contemplated before the first visit to the day hospital.
3. Consider referring the patient for day hospital attendance to assess Parkinson's disease and arthritis. Occupational and physiotherapy rehabilitation is aimed at improving gait, posture and mobility.
4. Try and persuade Mrs Smith to either:
   - (a) allow some furniture to be sold, and loose carpet fixed more firmly; have a commode; and get rails leading to and inside the toilet fitted by either the local authority or a private contractor after occupational therapy assessment; or
   - (b) again review with Mrs Smith the possibility of going into the more protected environment of a sheltered flat. If places are available, this is often more acceptable than trying to persuade someone against their will to go into a residential home. Alternatively, raise the possibility of the daughter coming to live with mother rather than the reverse.

Results

Unfortunately, none of the above suggestions bore fruit. Mrs Smith did attend day hospital, and was often seen to stumble, mainly due to a combination of poor gait related to her age and her osteoarthritic hips. When climbing stairs, however, it was noticed that she was particularly likely to be unsteady. Mrs Smith had worn bifocals for some years, so an ophthalmic review was requested because the lower part of bifocal spectacles are for near vision and stairs will appear out of focus; the patient may try to correct for this by altering his/her head position and thus disturb the balance. Trifocals are preferable – the middle part of these is for near vision, and both the upper and lower part of the lenses are for distant vision. Another tip is to check that spectacles are not dirty!

Even when using trifocals Mrs Smith was still unsteady. Although this was due mainly to the factors already described, there was no doubt that she was very anxious. Following a period of attendance at the day hospital for general 'rehabilitation exercises' Mrs Smith regained her confidence and her stability improved remarkably. Stopping the prochlorperazine she had been taking for some time for her 'dizziness' may also have helped, as this is one of several drugs that can aggravate or actually precipitate parkinsonian-type side-effects.

HOSPITAL, GENERAL PRACTITIONER, AND THE COMMUNITY

The assessment and diagnostic process, and the many possible lines of action and interaction, referral and management and supportive interplay between the hospital and its community are illustrated in Figures 7.1 and 7.2.

Figure 7.1 illustrates what might happen to the elderly victim of a fall or funny turn. She or he could remain at home, or be taken to the accident and emergency department, and then be sent home; or he or she might be admitted to almost any hospital department usually as an emergency, for investigation or treatment of an obvious underlying pathology or a complication such as a fracture, or because it is obvious or made obvious to the hospital that adverse social circumstances must preclude the sending home of the old person, at least without making better support arrangements. After investigation and treatment, including appropriate rehabilitation, often in a geriatric department, discharge home or sometimes to a home should usually be possible. Referral to the day hospital (from the general practitioner, from the accident and emergency department, or after a period of inpatient care) and a variety of clinical and social supports may all be required to minimize further episodes and reduce disability.

Figure 7.2 summarizes more specifically the interrelationships between the geriatric and other hospital departments, and the community generally.

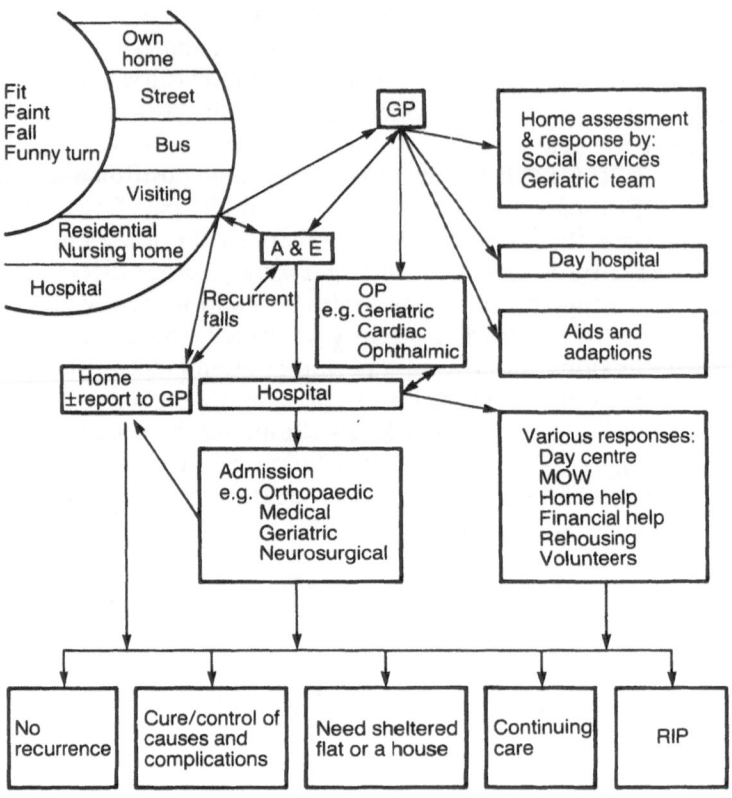

Figure 7.1 Hospital and community resources, their interfaces and interplay in the elderly with falls, faints, and funny turns

GENERAL COMMENTS ON TYPES OF FALL

The general circumstances and types of fall and other funny turns are dealt with in detail in other chapters, but several general aspects are worth highlighting. They help to clarify the circumstances in which these episodes are likely to occur and will therefore indicate the need for a certain pattern of response from either general practitioner or community or hospital or social services and, where appropriate, good liaison between the general practitioner and others in the community and the hospital. The generalizations all refer to falls, but of course falls are often the consequence of fits, faints and funny turns and many of these generalizations would apply to any funny turn in older people.

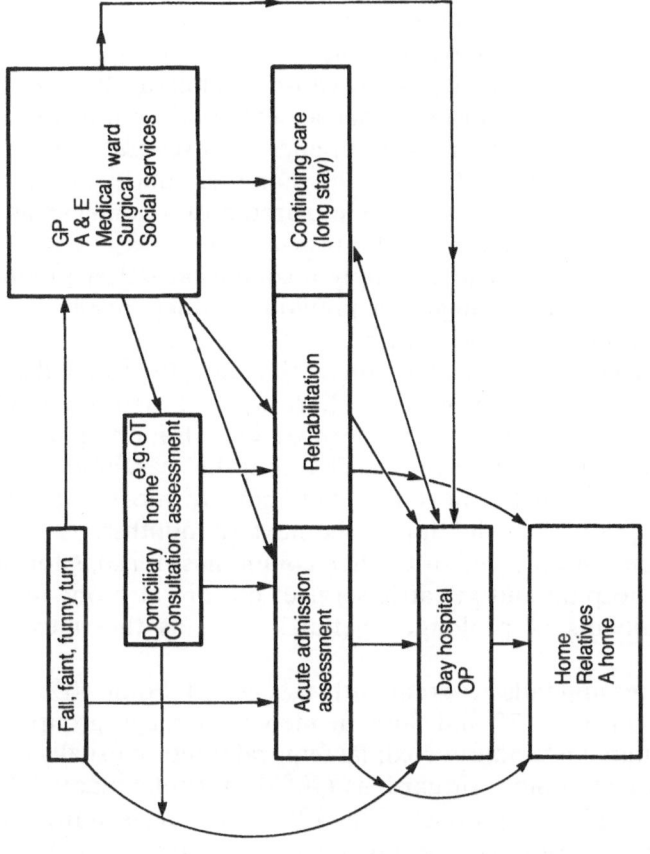

Figure 7.2 Falls, faints, funny turns and the geriatric services

1. Between a third and a half of falls are thought to be due to accidents and trips[1], often resulting from environmental hazards as well as partly from age-related defects in posture and gait[2,3]. There are many possible intrinsic medical causes such as osteoarthritis, parkinsonism, neurological apraxias, arrhythmias, poor eyesight and drug toxicity. Muscular weakness is often a factor.

   'Medical' falls are rather less likely to occur at night than falls in hospital, where they are often associated with the need to urinate, poor vision and impaired spatial perception in an unfamiliar and possibly inadequate environment, and less staff supervision.

   In many cases identifying the cause of a fall or other episode is not a question of diagnosing *either* an extrinsic *or* intrinsic cause but there is often a mixture of both and often several causes.

2. Women are far more likely to fall than men, partly because they are somewhat more likely to have impaired posture and gait as they age. Also, women are more likely to live alone[4].

3. Falls in the street usually imply a somewhat better prognosis than elsewhere as they suggest a previously independent or at least a more adventurous old person[5].

4. The longer the casualty has lain on the floor, the worse the prognosis in the long term as well as short term. Fractures, strokes, and coronaries as well as hypothermia, dehydration, pneumonia and pressure sores may develop. The 'long lie' casualties are not only more at risk in the next few days but are more likely than their contemporaries to die during the next 12 months[6].

5. Falls are not only one of the five commonest reasons for presenting to the hospital and geriatric service, but are also one of the major determinants of prolonged geriatric care as the outcome of the fall[7,8].

6. Fractures and falls are frequently associated. Some 40% of fractures in women over 75 and 30% in men in this age group have been precipitated by a fall[9]. Proximal femoral fracture usually occurs in or near private homes or gardens (70%) or public places (20%), only 10% being in institutions[10]. This 10% however, is in the 5% who are in these institutions. The greater frailty is not the only factor, and a hazardous environment, or staff shortages, may be other reasons.

7. Falls and fractures would seem to be more likely to occur in winter and during bad weather due to hazards outside the house and to the effects of significant reduction in temperature affecting mobility, cerebration, cardiac function and so on. There are two important consequences of this. The episode may lead to, as well as be caused by, hypothermia. Cold weather is associated with an increased risk of serious medical problems such as chest infection, myocardial

infarction, and stroke[11, 12]. These may precipitate or be the consequence of a funny turn, fall, etc.

8. Above all, falls are related to advancing age. The risk increases linearly in women so that 50% of those aged over 85 will fall. There is a similar, but less marked, rise in men up to the age of about 55; after that there is a drop in men, but not in the risk level for younger men. This is thought to be due to the survival of the substantially fit group of elite old men[9].

   If age *per se* is a marker of episodic disturbance then it will also reflect a likelihood of the victim having multiple medical, and social pathology as a context in which the management team will have to operate. Williamson *et al.*'s findings[13] of a substantial iceberg of unreported (and presumably unrecognized by the patient and previously unknown (to the general practitioner)) disabilities in old people has been confirmed many times. Of the substantially previously unknown disabilities 50% were amenable to at least some improvement, given appropriate treatment.

9. Not only are these turns likely to occur in the context of multiple pre-existing pathology not necessarily connected with the episode, but they are also themselves likely to be multifactorial rather than unifactorial. Falls etc. are likely to recur, and recurrent falls are particularly likely to be associated with medical pathology.

10. Surprisingly, few old people who fall actually need (ask for?) treatment. Although about one-third of the elderly fall at home during each year, some 2% require treatment[1]. In many cases, of course, people of any age are likely to be shaken up and bruised. However, it is surprising how often somebody who has been on the floor for a long time can get up, or be got up, and resume fairly normal activities almost immediately.

Overstall's[14] and Hamdy's[15] very helpful chapters on accidental falls are useful, informative reviews of this subject. Livesley's[16] succinct review suggests that unexpected, unexplained falls may often have a potentially remediable medical or environmental cause.

HOMEOSTATIC DYSFUNCTION AND DRUG TOXICITY

It is important both to the understanding and management of episodic disturbance in the elderly to appreciate the problem of age-related decline in homeostatic dysfunction. This may or may not be related to disease such as diabetes. Age differences are not the same as age changes.

The normal human body has a series of dynamically oscillating systems to maintain bodily equilibrium, for example in respect of balance and posture, gait, blood pressure, temperature, blood sugar and electrolyte levels. Disturbance of these homeostatic body-balancing functions may develop insidiously with advancing age but can be a potent cause of, or factor in, fits, faints, falls and funny turns. Even trivial environmental insults may be sufficient to make a slightly unstable old person trip up or fall over, particularly if they have other serious medical problems such as poor eyesight, or are taking drugs like hypotensives or hypoglycaemic agents which also affect one of these body-balancing systems. Pathological decline in the reserve of an organ due to unsuspected cardiovascular or cerebrovascular disease may further compound the problem and push an old person to the very brink of sudden collapse.

Diminished organ reserve, homeostatic defect, and pathology are all likely to be factors in the age-related risk of toxicity from excessive drug action, or drug side-effects or interaction. Ageing is associated with an increased risk of:

1. a diminished capacity to resist the drug's normal action without provoking excess effect;
2. diminished metabolism and clearance of drugs; and
3. the possibility of an increased sensitivity of target organs.

The accumulated pathology of old age often prompts polypharmacy and in addition the old person may buy medicines for themselves, so-called over-the-counter or OTC medication. This statistically increases the risk of side-effects and interactions.

Finally, the many other pathologies likely to be present in older people makes the body more susceptible to side-effects of the drugs and these side-effects are so often a cause of a fall or funny turn.

INFORMATION AND EDUCATION

The need for doctors, nurses, therapists, social workers and others dealing with elderly people to be fully acquainted with the circumstances of acute episodes, the patient's social background and what drugs they are on, cannot be repeated too often. The professionals and other carers – the elderly person, relatives, and volunteers – also need as much information as possible about what services are available and how to use them correctly: for example, when to ask for an acute admission; for the day hospital or day centre attendance; for home assessment by one of the geriatric team or domiciliary consultation for specific medical advice; for nurses, bath attendance, home helps or home care attendance; for luncheon clubs or meals-on-wheels; for drug information, etc.

Along with clinical care, administrative advocacy, and research (specially operational) the geriatric department must take on the main educational role in this area. The response to each patient referred to it, verbally or by letter is often educational. This should be complemented by a whole range of educational provision such as lectures, question-and-answer sessions, or tape and video presentations. Nowhere is this more important than in instructing the geriatric team (junior doctors, nurses, therapists, social workers) and hospital colleagues, the primary care team (general practitioner, nurses, social worker, home help and meals-on-wheels providers), the staff in homes and relatives and friends about disease, homeostatic dysfunction, drugs, and environmental hazards, than in respect of episodic dysequilibrium and altered consciousness.

Falls can often be found in the index or the main text in many geriatric textbooks and often 'rate' a whole chapter. However, it is remarkable how rarely fits, funny turns, or 'gone off' (feet or head) feature in many otherwise admirable books on geriatric medicine, and there is now a very substantial geriatric literature. Educating elderly people themselves and their immediate carers is also important. Practical demonstrations in the ward, rehabilitation areas or day hospital may be backed up by video records. Fear of falling can be a major disability in its own right, due to stroke[17], or to any of the many other destabilizing and weakening pathologies that can affect older people. This is not surprising as a fall could cause a potentially lethal fracture. In a stroke patient there is an above-average risk of a fracture because the bones on the affected side are likely to become osteoporotic. However, it is important to teach a scared old person and their relatives and friends that immobility can so easily lead to a downward spiral of deterioration, with balance, posture, coordination, gait, muscle power and blood pressure control all being affected. Muscular weakness and stiffness could very well contribute to further falls. Fear can actually increase spasm in a hemiplegic limb. Video can be used to educate fallers, and their relatives – including how to get up even if falls cannot be completely avoided.

Calculated risk-taking is as much a part of life for many old people and their relatives as for people of other ages. One could not and should not admit all old people at risk of falling, or those who have had a fall[18]. 'Blanket admissions' of all old people 'at risk' of falls and funny turns would deprive them of a deserved, albeit precarious, independent existence in their own home, quite apart from leading to collapse of the health service within a few days! Discussion of vulnerable old people's problems with their concerned carers is an important aspect of good geriatric care (see Case conference, p. 99).

THE GENERAL PRACTITIONER, ACCIDENT
AND EMERGENCY DEPARTMENT, MEDICAL
ADMISSIONS

All too often hospitals erect barriers to old people with falls and funny turns, especially if there is no obvious specific disease requiring admission such as stroke, complete heart block or a fracture. Even fractures, such as Colles, or a collapsed vertebral body, may not get them into hospital. The functional consequence of losing the use of an arm, or a painful back that may last for 5–6 weeks, can be very disabling. Some old people in this situation cannot be supported at home and will have to be admitted to a home or even to hospital. Confusion, whether or not due to dementia, is also likely to produce a resistance against finding a bed, whether or not there are physical problems.

One useful service is an overnight bed provision in the accident and emergency department. This allows time for an old person who is vaguely unwell, bruised, or confused, to be assessed, history obtained and suitable arrangements made for support and follow-up at home if he or she is not admitted. Assessment includes not only clinical observations and simple screening investigations such as blood counts, urea, electrolytes and electrocardiogram but also functional assessment by occupational or physiotherapists. This approach also gives social workers time to assess the situation. This arrangement will only work if the accident and emergency department is well supported by therapists and social workers and has good relationships with medical and social worker colleagues in the community. It also depends on collaboration with the geriatric and psychogeriatric colleagues in the hospital. It is essential for these two departments to have an effective presence in the main, i.e. DGH hospital where the casualty department is in terms of team input, as well as an adequate number of inpatient beds. Otherwise, the doctors and nurses in the casualty department tend to encounter the same barriers of which general practitioners so often complain.

There are probably two viable alternative methods of arranging medical admissions. They do not depend only on adequate numbers of medical, geriatric and psychogeriatric (and orthopaedic) beds but on a properly organized system of liaison between general practitioner, accident and emergency department, and the various hospital departments concerned:

(1) Obviously, surgical/orthopaedic patients are referred to the appropriate specialist on call. Clearcut or non-specific medical problems, whether they come direct from the general practitioner or via accident and emergency departments are separated on the basis of an age cutoff admission policy. In most hospitals a cutoff at 75 years has been used. In this system all medical admissions over 75 go into an acute admission assessment geriatric ward, and those under 75 are admitted by the medical

firm on take. There can be some flexibility in this system and some patients under 75 with 'geriatric' problems such as a stroke could be admitted direct to the geriatric department. Subsequent referral from surgical or medical wards to the geriatric department would follow the usual lines as shown in Figures 7.1 and 7.2, for example, for advice, or possible transfer for further assessment, rehabilitation or continuing care.

In this system, the majority of older people who present with fits, faints, funny turns and falls are likely to be admitted to the geriatric department initially which then takes on their ongoing care in terms of assessment, rehabilitation and discharge home where possible. As the geriatric department has a substantial 'presence' in the DGH it can provide an effective advisory role to other wards as well to the accident and emergency department. This should ensure that the geriatric medical care of elderly people who have been admitted to other wards, such as medical (for cardiac problems) or orthopaedic (for treatment of a fracture), is as good as possible, and where necessary colleagues in these other departments can ask for transfer at the appropriate time.

This pattern has been less clearly established in the field of psychogeriatric care but a similar approach of the presence of a team with some beds in the main hospital would help improve the care of the elderly people with confusional funny turns. Ideally, perhaps, all referrals of older people without clearcut medical problems, but whose obvious disability and illness seems to require admission, might come through a central department for the elderly with both medical and psychiatric staff.

(2) An alternative to this system is that all medical admissions come into the medical department on take. The senior staff in this department comprises at least two consultants. One has been trained in geriatric medicine, and the other is a general physician usually with a specific interest and training in some aspect of internal medicine such as cardiology. The geriatrician is then responsible for the special care of old people with geriatric problems and takes on an obligation to deal with their ongoing care whether it is organizing their discharge home or transferring them for further rehabilitation and, if necessary, continuing care.

In both systems the geriatrician and psychogeriatrician are also responsible for organizing day hospital care and liaising with the primary care team and the social services department to support old people who have had funny turns.

(3) Both these alternatives are infinitely preferable to the 'haphazard system'. In this so-called system a medical firm on take takes a substantial proportion of older people referred to hospital by a general practitioner or through the accident and emergency department whether they have specific or non-specific medical problems. The medical firm on take may or may not have a consultant-in-charge who has had training in geriatric medicine. The geriatric department in that district is on call all the time but

can only usually help with admissions if patients are referred directly to them, and of course if they have sufficient beds. As these beds are not always in the main hospital, the initial investigation of elderly people admitted to these beds may be difficult. Obviously, this approach is likely to lead to considerable friction between general practitioner and hospital, and between geriatrician and hospital colleagues.

The point has already been made that the problem of fits, faints, funny turns and falls is a reflection of the way we deal with the elderly generally and this is why the organization of the hospital – community interface in respect of admissions is not only a general problem but applies specifically to this aspect of geriatric care. Efficient organization of admissions will also carry with it the likelihood that referrals to outpatient departments such as ear, nose and throat for old people with disequilibrium, to cardiology for investigation of arrhythmias, to the psychiatric department for those with depression and dementia, and to the day hospital, are likely to be well organized. In some places local liaison has been rewarding, for example, the orthopaedic/geriatric liaison pioneered in Hastings (see Chapter 8). Recently, the technological advances in investigations such as the CT scan and NMR have also highlighted the need for good liaison between medical, geriatric, neurological and neurosurgical colleagues as well as with the accident and emergency department, for early investigation of old people with presentations that suggest a potential remediable cause for funny turns and falls.

The third edition of *Advanced Geriatric Medicine*[19] includes three interesting reviews of geriatric/orthopaedic liaison[20–23], preceded by an important section on the elderly in the accident and emergency department. Coakley's *Establishing a Geriatric Service*[23] also includes a chapter on geriatric orthopaedics from the pioneering Hastings department[24], and a synopsis of the various operational and admission policies to hospitals and to geriatric departments[25].

TAKING THE HISTORY

The general practitioner, family, friends and 'onlookers' should always try and identify, in as detailed a manner as possible, what led up to the turn and what were its clinical features. All too often the patient is referred to an outpatient clinic, the day hospital, for a domiciliary, to an accident and emergency department, or for an acute admission to a medical or surgical ward with either no details or only very few. 'Stroke, little stroke, recurrent stroke, transient ischaemic attack or funny turn' may be all that the referring doctor can truly identify as a provisional diagnosis; but these terms are often rather carelessly used, and the doctor should look really hard for important clinical features or possible causative factors including environmental hazards and potential drug side-effects that could at least have been mentioned. Nurses and staff in homes need to know about the problems of possible adverse drug side-effects and interactions.

The symptoms and signs of many problems in the elderly are often non-specific, and in the case of funny turns signs have often remitted by the time the general practitioner or hospital doctor arrives on the scene, but the patient, relatives and onlookers (including nurses) may have helpful information if questioned carefully. Home assessment to check on the environment and on the elderly person's functional capabilities in daily living activities are obviously likely to be important when there are repeated episodes/falls and no clear clues to their cause.

Drug-related Problems

A tabulation of known or suspected medical problems and drugs is vital and may give important clues. These may include, for example, diabetes: autonomic neuropathy, peripheral neuritis, or hypoglycaemia from insulin or oral agents; hypertension, ischaemic heart disease, heart failure: arrhythmias, and postural hypotension which may be due to drugs; gastrectomy, poor diet, being housebound: osteoporosis and osteomalacia (the latter may be associated with a myopathy), predisposition to fracture; syncope due to difficult micturition or defaecation; many drugs, especially those likely to cause psychomotor impairment (sedatives, tranquillizers, hypnotics, antidepressants), or hypoglycaemic and hypotensive agents, or diuretics, may be the cause of unsuspected postural hypotension. It is very important to prescribe and monitor medication carefully; for instance, L-dopa may reduce falls and funny turns by effectively treating Parkinson's disease, but it can cause toxic instability, arrhythmias or confusion. Problem-oriented records are very useful and can point to polypharmacy as a 'problem'.

Many other possible drug-related causes of funny turns could be described. Hypotensives and diuretics, used for hypertension or heart failure, L-dopa, and tricyclic antidepressants are all potent causes of postural hypotension, especially in an older person with cerebral or cardiac disease. Drugs that affect heart rate and output as well as cardiac rhythm should be suspected in patients suffering funny turns. Hypokalaemia causing tiredness and confusion as well as cardiac arrhythmias should be suspected in those taking diuretics, and/or having a poor diet, or taking excessive purgation. Other electrolyte and metabolic changes which are even less obvious can also be the cause of episodic disturbance. Hyponatraemia can occur with potassium-sparing diuretics such as amiloride, and also with chlorpropamide. Even with the best will in the world sensible old people may be taking many drugs, but may not be using them accurately.

Cardiac problems might recur because of both faulty compliance and interaction, lapses in thyroid medication could lead to a recrudescence of myxoedema, and previously well-controlled epilepsy might flare up again. Many psychotropic drugs such as sedatives, tranquillizers, hypnotics and mood controllers may cause episodic fluctuating confusion, hypotension, and falls, especially at night-time. Alcohol may do likewise, and the elderly are just as likely as younger people to imbibe alcohol excessively either as a long-term problem or as a recently acquired dependency, such as a response to bereavement.

WHERE THE EPISODE OCCURS

It may occur either in the home or in a public setting. If there are relatively few environmental hazards an intrinsic cause should be sought.

It has been suggested that environmental hazards inside and outside the home are overrated as a cause of falls and funny turns, as normal people have a great capacity for coping, usually subconsciously, with many dangerous challenges. However, even apparently trivial problems of uneven carpets, loose slip rugs, poor lighting, inadequate maintenance of damaged pavements, short pedestrian intervals on pelican-type crossings may be sufficient to cause trouble when intrinsic homeostatic dysfunction, definite pathology, or drug side-effects are present. The intrinsic problem may be more amenable to treatment, and if removed or minimized may abolish or substantially reduce the risk of subsequent attacks, even if environmental hazards remain.

A worrying aspect of falls is when they occur in a residential home or hospital. Keeping old people fit and mobile is very important – confinement to bed is bad – but slippery floors and confusing environments may lead to disorientation and dysequilibrium in institutions. Shortage of staff is sometimes highlighted as a problem in these days of financial restrictions, and certainly many residents in old peoples' homes tend to fall quite frequently. In a recent survey, more than half the residents had had one or more falls in a year; and a third of these had suffered significant injury as a result of the fall.

MANAGEMENT OF FALLS

The management of elderly people with fits, faints and falls can be broadly described in the following sequence, any part of which may involve the health or social services (and voluntary organizations):

1. Emergency action:
   (a) Pick or help them up, if there is no obvious serious injury.

(b) Contact their general practitioner.

(c) Dial 999 and arrange for them to go to hospital.

2. Treatment of any obvious cause, for example:
   (a) In their house – environmental hazards.
   (b) Footwear.
   (c) Poor eyesight, lighting.
   (d) Medical problems such as epilepsy, abnormal cardiac rhythm, postural hypotension, cervical spondylosis, transient ischaemic attack, Parkinson's disease, osteoarthritis.
   (e) Drug side-effects such as hypotension, hypoglycaemia, oversedation, excess alcohol.

3. Treatment of any complication, for example:
   (a) Of a fracture.
   (b) Of a facial or head injury, or a subdural haematoma.
   (c) Of the 'gone off their feet' syndrome because the old person is anxious or depressed.

4. Assessment and further investigation, for example:
   (a) Of (them in) their environment.
   (b) For possible hidden causes of syncope, dysequilibrium or muscular weakness.

5. Always try and record pertinent observations.

The episodes may have occurred in a house or flat, in the street, or an old peoples' home. They can, of course, also happen in a day hospital or ward. Only about 5% of the elderly are in homes or hospitals, so in most cases the starting point for the diagnostic/assessment/management process outlined in Figure 7.1 is community-based.

THE CASE CONFERENCE

A useful method of assessing old people who have suffered a funny turn, and of reviewing their progress, particularly with a view to discharge, is the case conference. The most important aspect of this team review is that it must allow all those present to make their point of view and to have it respected. The occupational therapist may feel, after a home assessment, that it is not possible or much too risky for an old person to return home at least for the time being. A similar point of view expressed by a patient or relatives must also be taken into consideration. At the same time, this type of meeting gives the geriatrician the opportunity to discuss with patients and their relatives, as well as community support personnel, just how much risk it is reasonable to take in allowing an old person to live at home rather than remain, dependent, in the hospital. It is important to bring both patients and relatives into the discussion and not leave them in an anteroom or in the ward, and one should not forget to invite the family doctor! It may also be useful to use a video recording to review progress and to demonstrate that an old person can get out of bed on his/her own, and can even get up off the floor after being put there as part of rehabilitation treatment.

Sadly, repeated case conferences, sometimes with video evidence, only confirm that the immobile or unstable or confused old person is static or even showing deterioration. In this situation it may be impossible to discharge the patient home again, although an alternative may be considered such as discharge to a relative or to a residential or nursing home.

PACEMAKERS

Episodic arrhythmias may cause faints, fits, funny turns, falls and fractures; these may be morbid or mortal.

The assessment, investigation and treatment of episodic disturbance of posture or consciousness for possibly treatable cardiac rhythm change is a prime example of liaison between patient, relatives, general practitioner, hospital departments (such as geriatric and cardiac), and bioengineers. Relatives are important here because they as much as the victim can help provide an accurate history of events by being advised to check on the pulse before, during and after 'attacks'; they may also be useful in elucidating the history of any funny turns.

Appropriate cardiac pacemaking may not only prevent unavoidable death from heart block and asystole, but it can also improve the quality of life of some old people, particularly those who have suffered cardiac attacks or who have heart failure or extreme fatigue. Many of these potential pacemaker recipients self-select, in that if they have extensive cardiovascular disease they will succumb to arrhythmias, heart failure or a coronary thrombosis. However, even though the prognosis is less good if there is obvious ischaemic heart disease or hypertension, a pacemaker is still indicated if this is symptomatic. The two main groups of elderly people who are now considered suitable recipients for pacemakers are those with complete heart block – virtually always symptomatic – and those with sinus bradycardia and sinoatrial disease (many of which are asymptomatic). This latter group tends to present at a somewhat younger age than those with complete heart block and the natural history is quite good. There should, therefore, be a higher threshold for implanting a pacemaker.

Combining the two groups, the current figures suggest that 70% of those in the 70–89 age group who receive a pacemaker are alive 5 years later.

This finding has put pressure on the pacemaker engineers to not only improve the general quality of the pacemakers, but to develop longer-life batteries; the model recommended by the DHSS in the past had a battery life of only 5–6 years so that most such patients required a second operation.

Continued work on pacemakers by bioengineers presents us with an increasing range of alternatives. For example, there are pacemakers that are rate-responsive and provide dual chamber pacing, rather than those that just respond from the right ventricular apex upwards such as life bundle branch block; pacemakers that respond to pH or lactic acid changes, or sense shortening of QT changes; single chamber pacemakers that are modulated by intercostal muscle function; tachycardia pacemakers with microprocessor memories to respond to a variety of stored memories of different tachyarrhythmias so that the paced patient is unaware of having an arrhythmia and does not experience a funny turn (this can be very useful in those who are insensitive to or suffer side-effects from antiarrhythmic drugs); and, finally, an implantable defibrillator, which though it cannot prevent the victim becoming unconscious for a short time, responds promptly by reviving him or her?

At a current cost of between £500 and £2000–£3000 for pacemakers, this treatment in appropriate elderly people can save life, and greatly improve the quality of life in those who are excessively tired of have heart failure, or in those who would otherwise suffer a fractured hip with its consequent morbidity and cost. Sadly, the current evidence suggests that the current rate of pacemaker implantation in the United Kingdom is approximately half of that recommended by the World Health Organization and considerably below that currently practised in most European countries. As far as one can judge this is not mainly due to financial restraints, but presumably rather to a lack of searching out and treating more people.

The starting point for assessment must obviously be a high index of suspicion, although a normal resting ECG should not include further investigation in suggestive circumstances, for example with a portable ECG tape, particularly one programmed to respond either to the patient's signal to start recording or to changes in rhythm or blood pressure. So-called diary ECGs are available.

One cautionary note should be sounded regarding patients suffering from dementia. While funny turns presenting as episodic confusion may very well be due to a potentially reversible underlying cause – whether cardiac arrhythmia, postural hypotension, vertebrobasilar insufficiency, cervical spondylosis or epilepsy – if there is sustained history of continued confusion it may be that the victim has irreversible dementia. It may still be worth pacing these people to prevent major complications such as fracture, but one should be extremely cautious about any prediction of improved cerebral functions. In the circumstances temporary pacing would be advised before implanting a permanent pacemaker.

An explanatory leaflet on pacemakers is issued by the British Heart Foundation[26]. There are now many useful pieces of literature from statutory or voluntary bodies such as the Parkinson's Disease and Alzheimer's Disease Societies, the British Diabetic Association, Age Concern and Help the Aged. We must also remember to explain to the victims of falls, faints and funny turns what has happened to them and how we are trying to prevent recurrence – far fewer old people are confused than we often seem to remember.

THE DAY HOSPITAL

The day hospital is a day-patient facility located within the geriatric department. Although there may be a hard core of dependent attenders who cannot be discharged unless an alternative such as a day centre is available, the day hospital should be distinguished from a social facility which provides mental and social stimulus, warmth and food, usually provided by a local authority or voluntary organization.

The day hospital has a substantial assessment and rehabilitation function, for example, for elderly people with arthritis, Parkinson's disease, stroke, or after fracture. In practice, the majority of old people who attend a day hospital come because of problems with mobility or stability, and it is only after a period of assessment that specific medical diagnosis and any homeostatic dysfunction is clearly identified.

Elderly people may attend a day hospital after a period of inpatient treatment in the geriatric or other department (orthopaedic, for instance), or attendance at the day hospital may avoid an inpatient admission. Although geriatric day hospitals are now regarded as an important part of a comprehensive geriatric service, the problems of transport to and from a day hospital may dominate efficient functioning. With good inpatient and outpatient investigation, and home and day care facilities, the actual need for specific day hospital provision may be reduced to between 15 and 20 places in an average-sized district.

Brocklehurst and Tucker[27] have published the definitive review of the functions and current situation regarding British day hospitals. Hildick-Smith[28] has recently pointed out that frequent day hospital attendance may actually be more costly than inpatient or residential alternatives, but is often preferred by the consumers/clients, and it is apparently staff-efficient (assuming that transport is effective). The oft-expressed confidence in the effectiveness of the day hospital in providing efficient patient care, and a good interface between hospital inpatient care and the local community, varies from district to district and with different stages in the evolution of a geriatric service[29-31].

RESEARCH AND RESOURCES

'Pure' clinical research is important in geriatric medicine, as already indicated in several of the references already listed. Another important example of screening in relation to falls, funny turns and fractures is the biochemical screening of unwell old people, for example, for various often unsuspected electrolyte metabolic disturbances such as hyponatraemia, thyroid disfunction, or osteomalacia, due to disease and/or drugs. Osteomalacia is associated with a myopathy that could lead to unstable gait and falls as well predisposing to fracture due to loss of bone strength. Biochemical disturbances can be a potent cause of psychological as well as physical turns.

It is important to remember that skill is often required when interpreting tests, and this underlies the need for geriatric expertise in providing laboratory and hospital services for family doctors and other members of the primary care team. For instance low protein levels often found in unwell old people could falsely distort tests and produce 'false positive' results. Another interesting aspect of this situation is that truly abnormal tests are misinterpreted. For instance, we have recently confirmed Ratcliffe's *et al.*'s finding[32]. After a stroke or accidental fall biochemical screening may reveal surprisingly severe muscle damage. Truly abnormal raised enzyme levels could be interpreted as always due to myocardial infarction. This, of course can be associated with a fall, and if relatively painless could only have been diagnosed by finding of raised 'cardiac' enzyme levels.

As well as the exciting area of clinical research it is important to pursue operational research. Effective and efficient hospital community responses, as indicated in Figures 7.1 and 7.2, depend on adequate provision of the right resources. An interesting survey of the present level of remedial therapists staffing in three-quarters of the departments of geriatric medicine in the United Kingdom[34] showed such a shortfall that it could not be explained entirely by a problem of underfinancing. There is clearly an acute shortage of therapists, and it is unrealistic to expect any new training colleges to be established within the next few years to meet this shortfall. Andrews and Brocklehurst[33] suggest the development of a new kind of training for rehabilitation nursing with its own post-basic qualification. These nurses would not replace the work of therapists, but would complement and supplement it.

What other initiatives might research or simple clinical observation suggest to help the elderly who are suffering funny turns? A vital area is the development of a home care team to support an elderly person in his/her own home, avoiding hospital admission, or to be brought into action to 'cover' a difficult discharge. The team could include a community nurse, occupational therapist, social worker, and home help, and liaison within the team would ensure that there was no unnecessary overlap or duplication, and that there was efficient monitoring of the situation. If and when the elderly person improves, the frequency of home help or meals-on-wheels provision or nurse visiting could be reduced, or possibly stopped altogether. A particularly important member of this home care team is the home help, and has been suggested that in the future the role of home help could be extended considerably. Given appropriate training at the time of appointment, and inservice educational support, there is no reason why a home care attendant could not do at least as much as a devoted relative, such as shopping, or collecting pensions; preparing and serving meals and even helping with feeding; helping with washing and dressing; cleaning around the house, and laying and lighting fires; laundry and even emptying commodes; and maybe even the administration of medicines in liaison with family doctor and community nurse. It is likely that many home helps already do many of these duties, but their terms of service in fact preclude them from undertaking them. It would be better to acknowledge the reality of the situation, by appropriate education and remuneration.

A major problem in this area is to bring to wider attention successful developments following operational research. Local experiments and successful innovations can be brought to a wider audience through educational meetings, by medical journals such as *Age and Ageing* and *Geriatric Medicine*, and publications such as Ferlie's *Source Book of Initiatives in the Community Care of the Elderly*[34], or regularly published copies of DHSS lists of selected important references.

Appropriate research may confirm or refute long-held beliefs. The correct way to approach the setting up of age/sex registers, and the choice of effective methods of screening of the at-risk elderly, are fascinating but as yet somewhat unresolved areas. High-powered research is probably not needed to justify designing ward and residential home environments to include good lighting, a choice of beds and chairs appropriate to the height of the elderly person using them, and the careful use of drugs including night sedation, but research *is* needed to confirm the hopes or benefits of assessment and intervention amongst the elderly. A recent survey[35] does seem to indicate that regular 'intervention' visiting followed by the provision of appropriate social/community or medical services (without any clinical examination being carried out by the surveying visitor) reduced the number of both emergency medical calls and admissions to hospital for the intervention group compared with the control group. The survey showed that subjects in the 'intervention group' benefited from the provision of aids and modifications to their homes, and from increased confidence as well as medical intervention where necessary.

The attendance allowance paid in the United Kingdom is an example of how financial help can be given to carers who look after the disabled for part or whole of the 24 hours. The number of allowances is increasing all the time, probably due to a combination of the increasing frailty of a minority of the very old and to a gradually increasing public awareness of the availability of this allowance. There was an increase of 17% in applications to the DHSS for the attendance allowance in the first 9 months of 1984. The payment to carers is for supervision of those *at risk* of falls faints and funny turns, as well as for physical care. It acknowledges the heavy commitment for devoted relatives and friends who may very well have had to give up work. In the 3 months July–September 1984, more than 13 000 of a total of just under 17 000 of newly awarded allowances at the higher rate were for the over-65s. More than 22 750 of around 29 250 new awards at the lower rate in this 3-month period were for the over 65s, who are still less than 20% of the total population; a substantial proportion of these awards are for those aged 75–90. The four main groups of disability meriting the granting of an allowance were those affecting the circulatory system, mental disorders, musculoskeletal system and connected tissue diseases, and diseases of the nervous systems and sense organs (Morris, personal communication).

CONCLUSION

The need for team work pivoting around the elderly victim of a fit, faint, fall or funny turn has been referred to several times in this chapter. The need for doctors, nurses, therapists, social workers and anyone dealing with elderly people to be fully acquainted with the circumstances of acute episodes, with patients' social background and what drugs they are on, cannot be repeated too often. The professionals and other carers – the elderly person, relatives, and volunteers – also need to be well informed about what services are available and how and when to use them, such as when to ask for an acute admission, a day hospital or a day centre attendance, or home assessment by any member of the geriatric care team or a specific domiciliary consultation for medical advice, for nurses, bath attendance, or home care attendance, or for luncheon clubs or meals-on-wheels, and for information from the local drug centres.

Many specific ways of abolishing or minimizing episodic disturbance in the elderly have been indicated in this and other chapters. In summary prevention can be by:

1. improving or training for a dangerous environment or changing the environment for somewhere else; and/or
2. dealing with intrinsic medical problems by appropriate treatment and careful, educated use of medication; and/or
3. preventive treatment (such as the use of aspirin in men who have suffered transient ischaemic attacks), or appropriate pacing for arrhythmias.

General, long-term prophylactic action based in general practice may be very helpful. These include: the use of age/sex registers to identify those most at risk because of multiple disabling pathology and adverse social circumstances; and screening, for example, eye, ear and foot problems. Referral to a chiropodist, for instance, may effect a miraculous cure!

References

1. Waller, J. A. (1976). Falls among the elderly – human and environmental factors. *Accident Analysis and Prevention.* This is a United States publication. Fuller references may be available.
2. Sheldon, J. H. (1960). On the natural history of falls in old age. *Br. Med. J.*, **5214**, 1685–90
3. Lucht, U. (1971). A prospective study of accidental falls and resulting injuries in the home among elderly people. *Acta Socio-Med. Scand.*, **2**, 105.
4. Overstall, P. W., Imms, F. J., Exton-Smith, A. N. and Johnson, A. L. (1977). Falls in the elderly related to postural imbalance. *Br. Med. J.*, **1**, 261.
5. Devas, M. B. and Irvine, R. E. (1969). The orthopaedic geriatric unit. *Br. J. Geriatr. Prac.*, **6**, 19
6. Wilde, D., Nayak, L. and Isaac, B. (1981). Facts on falling. *Hlth. Soc. Serv. J.*, **91**, 1413–15.
7. Naylor, R. and Rosin, A. J. (1970). Falling as a cause of admission to a geriatric unit. *Practitioner*, **205**, 72.
8. Isaacs, B., Livingstone, M. and Neville, Y. (1972). In *Survival of the Unfittest: A Study of Geriatric Patients in Glasgow*, p. 78. (London: Routledge and Kegan Paul).
9. Exton-Smith, A. N. (1977). Clinical manifestations. In *Care of the Elderly, Meeting the Challenge of Dependency.* p. 47 (Eds Exton-Smith, A. N. and Grimley Evans, J.) (London: Academic Press).
10. Brocklehurst, J. C., Exton-Smith, A. N., Lempert Barber, S. M., Hunt, L. and Palmer, M. (1976). Fracture of the femoral neck. *HMSO Report No 1 to the Department of Health and Social Security*, p. 71.
11. Bull, G. M., Brozovic, M. and Chakrabarti, R. (1979) Relationship of air temperature to various chemical, haematological and haemostatic variables. *J. Clin. Pathol.*, **32**, 16–20.
12. Keatinge, W. R., Coleshaw, S. R. K., Cotter, F., Mattock, M., Murphy, M. and Chelliah, R. (1984). Increases in platelet and red cell counts, blood viscosity, and arterial pressure during mild surface cooling: factors in mortality from coronary and cerebral thrombosis in winter. *Br. Med. J.*, **289**, 1408.
13. Williamson, J., Stokoe, I. H., Gray, S., Fisher, M., Smith, A., McGhee, A. and Stephenson, E. (1964). Old people at home – their unreported needs. *Lancet*, **1**, 1117–20.
14. Overstall, P. W. (1978). Falls in the elderly – epidemiology, aetiology and management. *Recent Advances in Geriatric Medicine* (ed. Isaacs, B.), p. 61–72. (Edinburgh: Churchill Livingstone).
15. Hamdy, R. C. (1984). Accidental falls. *Geriatric Medicine. A Problem-orientated Approach.* pp. 1–16. (London: Baillière-Tindall).
16. Livesley, B. (1984). Falls in older age. *Br. Med. J.*, **289**, 568
17. Richardson, A. (1959). *Never Say Die. A Return to Everyday Living for the Partly Disabled*, p. 41. (London: Max Parrish).
18. Boyd, R. V. (1981). What is a 'social problem' in geriatrics? *Health Care of the Elderly*, pp. 150–1. (ed. Arie, T). (London: Croom Helm).
19. Irvine, R. E. (1983). Geriatric orthopaedics at Hastings: the collaborative management of elderly women with fractured neck of femur. In *Advanced Geriatric Medicine* 3, pp. 130–6. (London: Pitman).
20. Burley, L. E. (1983). The joint geriatric orthopaedic service in South Edinburgh. *Advanced Geriatric Medicine 3*, p. 137–43. (London: Pitman).
21. Taggart, H. (1983). Geriatric-orthopaedic rehabilitation in Belfast. *Advanced Geriatric Medicine* 3, pp. 144–50. (London: Pitman).
22. Scott, P. J. W., Roberts, M. A., Auld, J. and McGregor, I. (1983). The use of an accident and emergency department by the elderly. *Advanced Geriatric Medicine* 3, pp. 125–9. (London: Pitman).

23. Coakley, D. (ed.) (1983). *Establishing a Geriatric Service.* (London: Croom Helm).
24. Irvine, R. E. (1982). A geriatric orthopaedic unit. In *Establishing a Geriatric Service*, pp. 166–80. (ed. Coakley, D.) (London: Croom Helm).
25. Pathy, J. (1982). Operational policies. In *Establishing a Geriatric Service*, p. 37. (ed. Coakley, D.) (London: Croom Helm).
26. British Heart Foundation (1983). *Pacemakers*, Heart Research Series No. 9.
27. Brocklehurst, J. C. and Tucker, J. S. (1980). *Progress in Geriatric Day Care.* King Edward's Hospital Fund for London.
28. Hildick-Smith, M. (1984). Geriatric day hospitals – changing emphasis in costs. *Age Ageing*, **13**, 95–100.
29. Anand, K. B., Thomas, J. H., Osborne, K. L. and Osmolski, R. (1982). Cost and effectiveness of a geriatric day hospital. *J. Roy. Coll. Physicians Lond.* **16**, pp. 53–6.
30. Tucker, M. A., Davison, J. G. and Ogle, S. J. (1984). Day hospital rehabilitation. Effectiveness and cost in the elderly: a randomised controlled trial. *Br. Med. J.*, **289**, 1209.
31. Murphy, P. and Rai, G. S. (1984). Pay hospital rehabilitation – effectiveness and cost. *Br. Med. J.*, **289**, 1541.
32. Ratcliffe, P. J., Ledingham, J. G. G., Berman, P., Wilcock, G. K. and Keenan, J. (1984). Rhabdomyolysis in elderly people after collapse. *Br. Med. J.*, **289**, 1877–8.
33. Andrews, K. and Brocklehurst, J. C. (1984). Provision of remedial therapists in geriatric medicine. *Br. Med. J.*, **289**, 661.
34. Ferlie, E. (1983). *Sourcebook of Initiatives in the Community Care of the Elderly. PSSRU* University of Kent.
35. Hendriksen, C., Lund, E. and Stromgard, E. (1984). Consequences of assessment and intervention among elderly people: a three-year randomised controlled trial. *Br. Med. J.*, **289**, 1522–4.

Further Reading

Age Concern Publications, including *Profiles of the Elderly, No. 5: Accidents* (1977).
Caird, F. I., Kennedy, R. D. and Williams, B. O. (1983). *Practical Rehabilitation of the Elderly.* (London: Pitman Medical).
Darnbrough, A. and Kinrade, D. (1979). *Directory for the Disabled*, 2nd Ed. (Cambridge: Woodhead Faulkner Ltd.).
Denham, M. J. (1983). *Care of the Long-Stay Elderly Patient.* (London: Croom Helm).
Hodkinson, H. M. (1976). *Common Symptoms of Disease in the Elderly.* (Oxford: Blackwell Scientific Publications).
Keeble, U. (1979). *Aids and Adaptations.* (London: Bedford Square Press).

8

After a Fall

K. G. F. BENTON and T. M. STROUTHIDIS

INTRODUCTION

The hospital and the community are so intimately related that a change in the one will eventually be reflected by a change in an aspect of the other. Although it may appear that to an orthopaedic surgeon a fall is of no apparent consequence unless it breaks a bone, the group most likely to fall and to break a bone from a fall is nevertheless expanding more rapidly in numbers than any other section of the population[1]. This means that each year there will be more patients with orthopaedic injuries including fractures of the proximal femur. There has in addition been a rapid growth of orthopaedic waiting lists for elective operations. The dilemma that falls have in part created for the surgeon then is the balance of emergency work against elective surgery and the reduction of the waiting time for elective orthopaedic operations[2].

The efficient mobilization and rehabilitation of elderly patients in orthopaedic beds has therefore become crucial to the provision of an effective orthopaedic service. However, old people undergoing rehabilitation from a fall, and this must include the repair of broken bones, are often beset by so many medical problems[3] that they need the attention of a physician skilled in geriatric medicine. The orthopaedic surgery on its own, no matter how good, is simply not enough and a system of collaborative care will be required between the orthopaedic surgeon and the physician in geriatric medicine. On the other hand to a physician dealing with elderly patients every fall is an affair of interest in itself, and the decline of an elderly person can often be clearly dated from such an event. A fall always happens for a reason and until proven otherwise every fall must be regarded as a symptom[4]. Often it is an expression of serious disease and the factors underlying its occurrence must be found and dealt with. The importance of viewing a fall as a symptom cannot be overstated, and the need to determine the cause of falling in every case of falls must not become obscured by the events to be described.

INJURIES AND SEQUELAE FROM FALLS

Falls in old age are well recognized as an important cause of serious morbidity and they will often have lethal complications[5]. Even though an isolated incident with no obvious cause or effect may soon be forgotten or regarded as negligible, many of those who fall will be liable to do so again[6]. The majority of falls occur inside the home, and do not usually harm the fallers or lead to medical advice, but most fatal home accidents are due to falls. Indeed, more old people die from accidents in the home than the entire number killed on the roads each year[7]; women are the victims at least twice as often as men, a difference that has been attributed to the stepping pattern of the female gait[8]. The proportion of all falls complicated by physical injury is actually less than one-quarter, and the majority of falls do not break bones, but the overall number of injuries requiring medical attention is enormous because over one-third of the elderly population fall each year. Although much interest has focused on fractures of the femoral neck resulting from falls in old age, in fact fewer than one in every 100 women who fall will sustain a fractured neck of femur[9], but falls will cause many other problems apart from fractures.

Very often the worst and most protracted effect of falling is fear and loss of confidence, and any failure to determine the cause of falls will result in a vicious circle and an early repetition of events. Fear will restrict social mobility, generate anxiety in the carers and severely limit the activity of the fallers. Indeed an elderly person may be so frightened after a fall that he or she may refuse to rise from a hospital chair or may feel no longer able to live alone. This is a serious state of affairs which has been referred to as the 'post-fall syndrome', and although it may represent a pathological phobia[10] it may also result from a disturbance or misinterpretation of sensory information in those who have lost their sense of what is vertical. Each day in this country over 100 old people will lie on the floor all night after a fall from which they cannot rise. Low environmental temperatures and impaired physiological responses to cold put these people at great risk of hypothermia, especially when the fall is associated with postural hypotension or night sedation, and this includes alcohol. Cuts and bruises around the face are very common complications of falls and they may occasionally cause eating problems. Furthermore, many patients who are admitted to hospital because of a fall have pneumonia and dehydration and a few who fall will develop a subdural haematoma. These complications may both precede and cause the final episode in a cluster of falls as premonitory and terminal events[11]. Generally around one in ten falls will result in a fracture even though most falls are not likely to cause physical damage warranting medical attention. It follows that falls in old people which cause physical harm will often break bones. The main reasons which underlie this commonsense fact are: first, the high incidence of skeletal fragility resulting from the osteoporosis that comes with old age; and, second, the impairment of automatic reflexes which might otherwise prevent a heavy fall. Osteoporosis and impaired righting reflexes will also influence the frequency with which certain types of fracture are seen.

Overall, one of the commonest fractures found in old people examined after falling down is a Colles fracture of the wrist and, as with other fractures, its pattern of incidence has a marked change with age[12]. In young people wrist fractures are commoner in men than in women and they usually result from direct violence outside the home. However, in old people this pattern is reversed so that in the elderly most fractures are seen much more often in women, and they invariably result from accidents, usually falls occurring inside the home. The Colles fracture provides an excellent example of a fracture pattern that demonstrates a dramatic change with age. This fracture shows two age-related peaks of incidence (Figure 8.1). The first peak occurs in early adult life at about 20 years of age and is small. It contains more men than women, and thereafter only a gradual increase in the fracture rate for men is seen throughout life. The second and by far the greater of the two peaks is seen at the onset of old age but it has an overwhelming preponderance of women, for whom the fracture rate has now increased tenfold. Furthermore it is known that the most rapid loss of bone in women occurs within 10 years of the menopause, whereas bone loss in men occurs much more gradually. Hence the most reasonable explanation for the rapid rise in Colles fracture rate in women but not men is their inferior bone status at the time of falling, compared with their premenopausal state.

The situation for fractured neck of femur is different. There is still a marked change in fracture pattern with ageing but this affects men as well as women (Figure 8.2). In both sexes, after a small peak in early adult life at around 20 years of age, the fracture rate remains small below the age of 60 years and then it increases exponentially with age. Eventually, in old age, at around 75 years, fractures of the femoral neck become more common than fractures of the wrist. Indeed the rate of incidence of fractured neck of femur will double every 5 years in women and every 7 years in men[13]. The rise in fracture rate with age depends on the amount of bone present at the time trauma is sustained, compared with the amount of bone that was present in earlier life. That is to say the likelihood of a

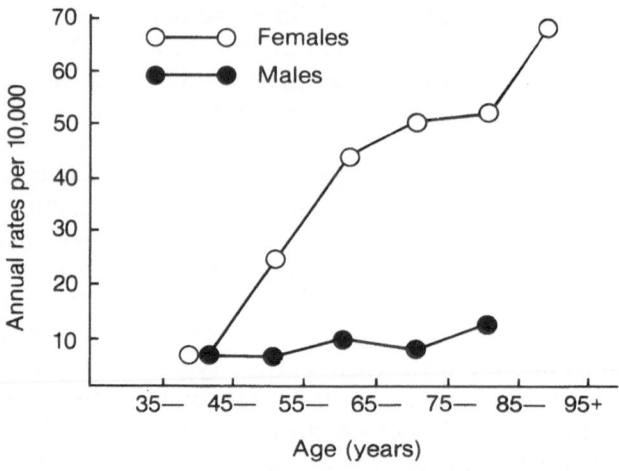

Figure 8.1   Colles fracture (reproduced by kind permission of Professor Exton-Smith)

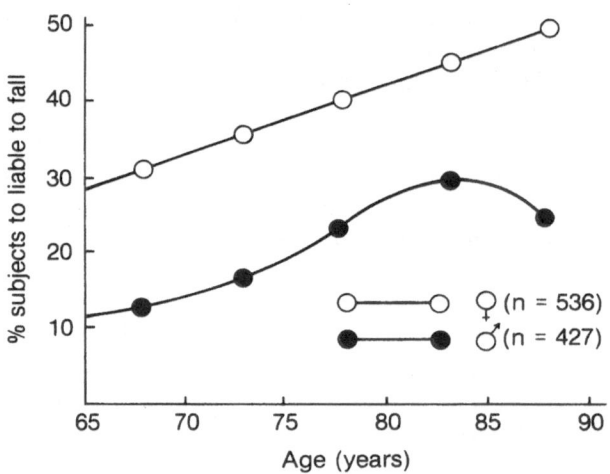

Figure 8.2   Age incidence of falls (reproduced by kind permission of Professor Exton-Smith)

person sustaining a fracture as a result of a fall will depend upon the amount of bone that has been lost overall.

This then explains why a fracture is more likely to complicate a fall in an older individual, but it does not account for the rate of rise of fractured neck of femur exceeding that of the wrist as age advances. One possible explanation of this phenomenon is that the reflex-correcting mechanisms are more likely to be impaired in the older patients so that when they fall there is no protection from the automatic stretch reflex of putting out their hand, and consequently the brunt of the injury is taken by the hip.

Clearly falls in old age are an abiding menace and indeed for many who do not avoid them, these everyday happenings are often a predictor of forthcoming death. Falls which lead to a fractured neck of femur as well as those which do not will carry a high mortality[14]. At least one-quarter of all old people who fall inside their homes will be dead within a year. The more housebound an old person is before the fall, and the longer the time spent unattended on the floor, the worse the prognosis seems to be. This appears to reflect the gravity of the illness responsible for the fall and the severity of the trauma sustained[15] rather than the circumstances in which the faller lives. Furthermore, it seems to be the complications of falling rather than the falls themselves which are likely to be brought to the notice of the general practitioner or a hospital department.

THE CASUALTY DEPARTMENT

For many elderly people the casualty department is a gateway to treatment for the injuries and illnesses that may attend their falls. It provides quick and easy access to medical care for all comers because referral by a doctor is not required first. Although it does not have a primary concern for inpatient care it is able instead to seek opinion from and refer for admission to all other hospital departments at any time of day. To the general practitioner seeing those who fall at home a casualty department is the normal source of help in treating minor injuries and assessing other trauma, but it also caters for those who have fallen in the street and for those sent in through the emergency services by relatives and friends. It is first important, however, for everyone who may attend an elderly patient at the scene of a fall not be misled by an *absence* of pain and the *presence* of mental confusion. Pain in the elderly will frequently result in mental confusion[16], and old people will often endure painful conditions without complaint but they will usually then admit to pain if asked direct. In general also there is little virtue in an urgent rush to hospital and, especially when a fracture is suspected, the interests of the elderly will be better served by a gentle ride in the ambulance and by a minimum of painful jolts. The first concern of the nursing staff in a casualty department after the arrival of an elderly patient will be to comfort the patient at a time of personal crisis and to prepare him/her for an initial evaluation of injuries and illness.

All elderly patients brought in as emergencies to a casualty department should be fully undressed before a medical examination, because otherwise injuries may be missed and clues to the patient's level of functional independence that preceded the fall will be lost. It is during this preparatory phase that hypothermia is often first suspected and that attention is directed to the patient's skin. It is essential in every elderly patient to prevent pressure on the skin from contact with hard surfaces as soon as possible. Thick plastic foam which is carried in the ambulance should always be placed under the sacrum and the heels as soon as the patient is put onto a stretcher. These sponge pads must remain in position until the patient can be transferred to a suitable mattress in a hospital ward or until the patient is again mobile. Prevention is by far the best treatment of pressure sores but this is difficult to achieve in practice because even where a pressure sore is not yet evident it may well be that damage has already been done to the skin during the period of immobility that must exist between the occurrence of the fall and the intervention of preventive nursing. Despite measures to prevent them superficial pressure sores will still develop in over one-third of all patients with fractures of the proximal femur, and the much more serious deep sacral sore is said to occur in about 10% of these patients.

Once the patient has been correctly prepared a full examination is carried out and often several coexisting conditions will be found and immediate treatment may be needed for some. Every old person presenting with an impairment of consciousness following a fall requires a prompt exclusion of hypoglycaemia by an estimation (by Dextrostix) of the plasma glucose concentration. Obviously the primary management of fractures and resuscitation from cardiorespiratory illness or blood loss are bound to take priority over a determined investigation into the cause of the fall, but this must be made at an appropriate time. Internal injuries which require surgical intervention are very uncommon after a fall and subdural haematomata do not tend to be acute complications, partly because in elderly people the intracranial dura is often adherent to the pia mater, but also because acute forms of intracranial bleeding in proximity to the dura are likely to be fatal before any means of intervention are at hand. Soft tissue trauma, usually cuts and bruises, will normally be dealt with last and this must include a review of tetanus immunity in every such case.

The identification of bony injuries in elderly fallers is made very much easier by their propensity to bruise. Nevertheless, there is generally a large demand for radiographs to examine elderly subjects, reflecting a high expectation of fractures in elderly patients. Several studies from casualty departments report that up to one-quarter of all elderly patients seen after falling down will be submitted for plain radiography, but only about a quarter of these will yield positive results[17]. On clinical grounds alone a diagnosis of bony injury to the shoulder girdle and upper limb can often be made with certainty because deformity and crepitus in this region are generally fairly obvious.

Fractures of the hip are much more difficult and they are by no means always associated with external rotation and shortening of the affected limb. Many old people have pain in the region of the hip following a fall but without evidence of deformity and their radiographs demonstrate osteoarthrosis as the only abnormality. Provided that these patients can weight-bear and walk a few unassisted steps in the casulty department they can usually be discharged to the care of their general practitioner as long as they are judged to be safe and to have a suitable home. Some such patients, however, are unable to weight-bear despite a normal radiograph taken shortly after injury, and these patients will need admission to hospital for mobilization and further observation. A few days later the radiographs will be repeated in some of these patients because of continuing pain and a general lack of progress and the disimpacted femoral fracture will then be clearly seen. Nevertheless, the possibility of pathological fractures, osteomalacia and, in active old people, fracture due to simple stress resulting in a fall must always be considered and therefore it is important to determine whether pain was present at the site of fracture, but before the fall occurred.

Finally, the opportunity should never be missed in the casualty department to establish the circumstances of the fall by information obtained from the ambulance crew, the referral letter from the general practitioner, and above all the relatives and friends or the nursing staff in residential homes if they accompany the patient to the hospital. These various sources of information are invaluable in offsetting a lack of clarity in the elderly patient's account of a fall given shortly after injury. All too often old people are sent straight home from a casualty department after presenting with falls simply because there is insufficient injury to warrant admission. Many of these patients have unsuitable homes, and there is a clinical impression that they suffer repeated falls and will not, unfortunately, be brought to the attention of the general practitioner before their functional capabilities are seriously impaired. The further management of an elderly patient can only be planned after an assessment of his/her level of function and social circumstances has been made and very occasionally it will be found to preclude an immediate return home. Especially when referral cannot be made direct to the geriatric day unit, the reason for the patient's visit to a casualty department should always be communicated to the general practitioner before the patient is finally discharged from the hospital.

RESUSCITATION AFTER FALLS

Acutely ill old people often respond well to intensive treatment and, except when death seems inevitable, energetic resuscitation may be needed for some. The main aim of resuscitation is to ensure an efficient circulation of an adequate volume of oxygenated blood at the correct temperature. Oxygen is usually readily to hand and is easy to administer, and following a fall it may be given at any time of circulatory collapse or respiratory failure including that caused by drugs. It should always be humidified and warm because the elderly are very prone to form mucus crusts. Upon arrival at the hospital a check must always be made for hypothermia as part of the routine nursing observations of an elderly patient. Prior to this, common-sense use will usually have been made of spare blankets and aluminium foil carried in the ambulance, but blankets and clothing should not be wrapped so tightly as to interfere with respiration in the exceptionally frail. Whenever the external body temperature fails to register in the lower reaches of an ordinary thermometer it is mandatory to establish the internal body temperature by means of a low reading thermometer placed in the rectum or vagina. If hypothermia (body core temperature less than 35.5 °C) is confirmed, the core temperature should be allowed to rise by means of passive reheating in a warm environment, at a rate not exceeding 1 °C per hour, and all forms of active interference must be kept to a minimum.

In elderly patients admitted in emergency following a fall dehydration is very commonly seen. The oral intake of food and drink should be encouraged as early as possible unless it is precluded by a stroke or loss of consciousness or the need for early general anaesthesia to manipulate a minor fracture. Those fractures which require internal fixation may not be operated upon until the following day and food and drink will need to be stopped only over 4 hours prior to the induction of general anaesthesia. When, however, dehydration is severe parenteral fluids are the treatment of choice. A dextrose solution (5%) is not the elixir of life, and wherever hypovolaemia is suspected normal saline should be carefully given until the extracellular fluid volume is replete. Every old person with a femoral fracture or with hypovolaemia must have an efficient cannula placed in a vein and sited to avoid the need for splinting the elbow or wrist. Some patients will eventually require a blood transfusion to replace the protein and red cell mass that is lost by sequestration at the site of wounds over several days. In practice, very few patients with fracture of the femur remain undiscovered for that length of time, and indeed most will have their fracture operated upon within the succeeding day. However, any pre-existing anaemia or blood loss which is not corrected during the period of operation may hinder the patient's rehabilitation. Therefore elderly patients with fracture of the femur should have blood samples taken when the drip cannula is placed in the vein. Blood may then be crossmatched for use if required, baseline estimations are made of the haemoglobin and electrolyte concentrations and a sample is saved for any retrospective measurement that may be indicated in the pretransfusion blood. Finally, the preliminary treatment of cardiorespiratory failure or the complications of diabetes mellitus is given where required on an individual basis.

HOME OR HOSPITAL?

It has already been mentioned that elderly patients presenting with falls should not be discharged straight away from emergency departments without suitable arrangements where these are indicated to further their care. It is just as important, however, that old people are not admitted to hospital purely on the grounds of age alone. The proper indication for admission after a fall is a complete loss of independence[18] on account of injury or illness which cannot be remedied on the spot. A partial loss of functional ability can often be compensated by suitable domiciliary support while treatment is continued on an outpatient basis. Thus any severe fracture which requires internal fixation to restore function is a clear indication for admission to an orthopaedic unit.

Equally, a fall caused by serious medical illness such as cardiac failure or stroke is also a reason for admission to an acute ward, preferably on the geriatric unit. In the event of serious illness and injury coexisting, and this is frequently the case – for example, the old person who falls and breaks a femur and then develops pneumonia while lying on the floor – rehabilitation cannot begin until function is restored by fixation of the fracture. There will then be little point in admitting such patients direct to an acute geriatric ward. The proper course should ideally be to admit to an orthopaedic bed and to improve the patient's condition with the assistance of the physician in geriatric medicine so that operation may be undertaken the following day. Sometimes the orthopaedic injuries may not be severe and the treatment is expectant, but the elderly patient with a fractured pelvis or vertebral body will often be effectively immobilized by pain. They will then require a level of support that is often best provided in a hospital environment, so they should be admitted, preferably to a geriatric unit, until their former independence is regained.

On the other hand a misplaced feeling of pity must not cause a patient to be unnecessarily detained in hospital. Occasionally, as after a head injury with transient loss of consciousness from an accidental fall all that is required is a period of careful clinical observation. Furthermore when a fall is associated with just a partial loss of functional capability it is often in an elderly patient's best interest to be managed and supported in the community, and indeed the majority will prefer it. Hence the active old person leading an independent life, and then suffering a truly accidental fall resulting in a minor fracture, will clearly not need to have his/her home life interrupted. Once the fracture has been manipulated under general anaesthesia he/she will be able to return home and still continue to receive intensive treatment at the fracture clinic. Indeed many old people who fall down on account of undefined chronic illness are often able to return to their own environment if they are supported by relatives and helpful neighbours, or if they live in a form of residential care. Their general practitioner is able and should be willing to undertake investigations into the cause of falling and to advise on the need for further domiciliary services as required, provided of course that he is first informed of a fall taking place. In this way, the failing and aged person with an unexplained fall may be maintained at home until further investigation and treatment such as that available in the geriatric day hospital, either restores independence or indicates that resettlement will be needed in the very near future.

Therefore, an accurate assessment of an old person's background and the circumstances in which he/she lives is essential if he/she is to remain at home after a fall or is to be discharged from a casualty department. It will then be necessary to first have a clear picture of what is needed for that particular patient to live in his/her own environment, and then to make arrangements for an appropriate level of support determined by individual needs. It is also vital to learn how the patient has been living in order to determine a decline of function since the onset of the falls.

However, old people frequently display an independent spirit and will often present a more optimistic account of their social circumstances and daily activities than is the actual case[19], so whenever possible their account must be balanced by the invaluable information that may often be obtained from the ambulance crew or general practitioner and from a discussion with the patient's relatives. The expressed wish of an elderly patient to return to their own environment without delay will frequently conflict with the needs of their family who may feel daunted by the prospect of continuing their support without interruption for a failing old person. Therefore, should any serious doubts remain about an elderly patient's capacity to be supported at home then admission to hospital will often be the wisest course. Otherwise every old person sent home from a hospital department after an unexplained fall must always be brought to the notice of his/her general practitioner, for whom there is available a wide range of options for investigation outside hospital, and these include referral to the geriatric day hospital when further assessment and rehabilitation is required.

THE GERIATRIC UNIT

It is estimated for this country as a whole that some 3 million elderly people fall each year[20] and so it should not be unexpected that falls are one of the commonest reasons for admission to a geriatric unit which directly accepts acutely ill patients. A few patients will then be referred to the geriatric unit from the casualty department after the exclusion of serious injuries, but most patients will be admitted as emergencies direct from home at the request of the general practitioner. Many geriatric units have now moved away from a traditional role of caring for the chronic sick in favour of an amalgamation of acute general medical wards for the elderly and a rehabilitation unit. Acute illness such as that presenting with a fall will then be managed in an atmosphere of rehabilitation and any treatment which does not in some way contribute to mobility will either be reconsidered or discarded, except when it is relevant to the terminally ill.

However, for the elderly patient in the geriatric unit, an emphasis on the management of acute illness will then create the same problems as are common among patients admitted under the other acute specialties. There are many forms of distress associated with inpatient care but the elderly tend to stay in hospital longer, are usually less articulate and always more vulnerable[21]. No matter how well they may conceal it and irrespective of their age, most patients are apprehensive during the first days of their stay on a hospital ward. Apart from being overrun by illness the elderly patient suffers a dramatic change in lifestyle and an altered timetable for the entire day. The routine that is required to keep the ward running well demands that patients must comply with the needs of the group[21], and so their identity as an individual is threatened. Patients may feel that their person is no longer of importance, a feeling that may have already have been engendered by their designation as a 'geriatric' patient. There are also the problems of noise and insufficient sleep[23], and of food that may not be entirely to an individual's liking. In addition the geriatric unit is a fearful place at night and night staff are never available in more than minimum numbers. Furthermore, the mentally intact may have a dread of enforced association with those who are confused or aggressive or seriously ill, and the social value of other ill people may not be readily appreciated by an individual patient. All this is endured because of a loss of independence, and reactive mental illness is common[24]. Every person's needs are individual and different irrespective of their age, and a particular quality manifest in geriatric nursing is a willingness to understand an old person's needs and a readiness to try and meet them.

It is clear that maintaining the identity of an elderly patient in a geriatric unit and preserving his/her personality is a matter of great importance. Nevertheless there is an equally fundamental need for accurate diagnosis and effective treatment of the physical and mental disorders that may have resulted in the fall. Illness in the elderly is very complex, and indeed several major disorders will often coexist in any one patient whose admission has resulted from falls. Several entirely separate skills will be necessary for its management, therefore the geriatric unit must function as a team under the coordination and leadership of a physician. The recognition of the fact that each member of the team imparts a contribution which no one else can make, and that no one contribution is all-important in the overall care of the patient, will enhance the therapeutic effectiveness and the job satisfaction of all those involved. A combined effort by all the members of the multidisciplinary team must then be directed at restoring as much mobility and independence as it is reasonable to obtain in any individual patient.

Often, however, rehabilitation will not be achieved without taking calculated risks such as walking on the stairs or practice in the kitchen, but these risks are taken in a supervised environment which by virtue of careful planning must not expose the patient to unnecessary danger. Apart from cross-infection and iatrogenic complications as many as one-quarter of all elderly patients may suffer an accidental fall during their stay on the ward[25] and some of these patients will sustain a fractured neck of femur. These falls are associated with patient activity such as getting out of bed or walking to the toilet, and seem to be an indication that rehabilitation is actually taking place. There is no great incidence of these falls when the nursing staff are depleted in numbers at night, but rather the falls serve as a reminder that any place of care can always be made safer by means of careful planning and design.

Lastly an essential part of rehabilitation consists of maintaining an elderly patient's grip on the outside world and this must require the promotion of the maximum amount of contact with the patient's family. In practice, it is usually very difficult to consider any patient without thinking about his/her relatives as well, and it is a vital part of care to appreciate the needs of the relatives and accept that sometimes their needs will inevitably conflict with those of the patient or the staff. It is well worth remembering that in liaison with the social worker the relatives will often play an essential part in the main aim of treatment, which must be a safe and planned discharge of the elderly patient back to the community, and an early return to the care of the general practitioner.

MEDICAL ASSESSMENT

The profound importance of accurate diagnosis of the physical and mental disease presenting with falls cannot be overemphasized. It is valid at all times, even in the very frail and it is fundamental to the patient's needs. In elderly people there are frequent reasons for falling which are directly related to age but the changes that precede these falls are not well understood. In general, the diagnosis will then be a matter of conjecture because usually there are several unknown coexistent aetiologies but with a final factor, which may be discernible and sometimes remediable, acting as the last straw. There are, however, many other causes of falling in the elderly but these causes are common to all age groups and they usually

result from well-defined and often treatable disease. It is now clearly
recognized that the elucidation of the cause of falling in the elderly is most
likely to succeed when it is undertaken as an exercise in general medicine[26].

TAKING THE HISTORY

The history is usually a helpful factor in determining the cause of a fall and
a method of matching a carefully taken history against a simple classification of the various kinds of fall has much to recommend it for the clinician.
Four categories of falls have been proposed[27]: and they are

1. accidental falls;
2. falls with loss of balance;
3. drop attacks or falls while walking;
4. falls or collapse with loss of consciousness.

These descriptive terms are somewhat imprecise because they are
limited by the language, but with the exception of accidental falls they are
not intended to make assumptions about the causes of a fall. They do,
nevertheless, allow an association with the fall to be identified around
which the history can be moulded. It is entirely accepted that different
conditions may be included in each of the particular categories of falls, and
that the various causes of falling may contribute to any kind of fall. In
practice, however, the history will usually be limited by the faller often
being the only source of information about a momentary and unexpected
event, and moreover repeated interrogation may result in a consistent but
not necessarily accurate story[28].

It has been pointed out that the difficulties the faller may have in putting
into words the experience of falling[29] can easily lead to errors in interpretation. An important study of falls inside the home[30] found discrepancies
between the fallers' response to the instruction 'Tell me what happened
when you fell?' and to direct questions such as 'Did you feel dizzy?' In this
study the fallers' own description of their fall rarely mentioned specific
symptoms, for example dizziness and lightheadedness, but instead tended
to convey the unexpectedness of the fall with no spontaneous recollection
of external hazards or associated symptoms. It was further pointed out that
when the patient suffers a truly accidental fall he/she is sometimes able to
definitely say 'I tripped up', and may then have a clear recollection of the
event. On the other hand 'I must have tripped', is better interpreted until
proved otherwise as '*I suppose* I must have tripped' really meaning
'Something happened which I can't explain and because I fell, I suppose I
must have tripped'. It is then sometimes revealing to ask the faller how
he/she tried to get up from the floor.

Furthermore, it is not uncommon for over one-half of elderly people in a general practice population to have experienced the subjective sensation described as dizziness[31]. This symptom is, however, rarely volunteered in spontaneous descriptions of falling given by the faller and tends instead to be produced in response to direct questions. It also correlates highly with evidence of psychosomatic disorders and with cerebrovascular rather than aural disease[32]. Therefore, unless dizziness is clearly associated with a change in hearing such as tinnitus and deafness preceding the fall, the temptation to medicate the vestibular apparatus should be resisted until the dizziness can be definitely equated with labyrinthine vertigo.

Lastly, a careful review of drugs is of particular importance in every case of falls. Special attention should be paid to over-the-counter products and this includes alcohol. The drug history will often point to previous diagnoses such as hypertension, and conditions which may contribute to instability such as Parkinson's disease. The elderly are at special risk of falls caused by hypertension that is overmedicated according to geriatric standards, and antihypertensive medication must be viewed with great suspicion. Finally, when mental impairment is present the history will often be less valid, but it is still well worth making an attempt to get an account from the patient. Sometimes a reasonable opinion can still be formed concerning the significance of any symptoms that are given, but inevitably a greater emphasis must be placed on questioning those who may have witnessed the fall, if indeed any witnesses are available.

CLINICAL EXAMINATION

The presence of mental impairment will impose a greater reliance on the clinical examination. This demands an attention to detail and it must highlight the special features of relevance to falls in an elderly patient. An assessment of the mental state is an indispensable part of the examination of every old person[33]. Its importance may be judged from the fact that over half of the patients admitted to an acute geriatric ward have some degree of brain failure. When it persists, brain failure will make it difficult for the patient to be rehabilitated and it is associated with a shortened life. Anxiety and depression are also very common in the elderly population but they are much harder than brain failure to detect. Early morning waking, for instance, is an unreliable sign in the elderly because many old people wake up several times at night. The more usual features are agitation or apathy and a preoccupation with physical complaints. Many elderly people live alone, isolated and housebound with friends or relatives far away or dead. They have few stimuli and cannot afford or have not the patience or ability to watch television, listen to the radio or read[34]. It is therefore most important to determine if they still find life worth living even though most have little prospect of an improvement in their lives.

Emotional disorders and brain failure will decrease the capacity for alertness, motivation for rehabilitation and self-care, and combined with other diseases will lead to confusion, apathy or wandering and may eventually result in falls. Nevertheless, any disorder in the special senses may well be remediable, and can help make a patient's life better and safer. Visual input is very important in controlling postural sway, and both poor eyesight and impaired hearing will contribute to the risk of isolation and falls. Visual impairment may be the result of disease and deterioration of the retina and lens, but may also be the result of not cleaning and not possessing or failing to wear spectacles. In every case the spectacles should be checked because those which were suitable many years ago may still be worn, despite a marked deterioration in the lens. Careful fundoscopy and measurement of the visual acuity should be routinely undertaken on the ward. A patient's hearing aid should also be in working order so that everything is done to maintain communication.

The elderly will frequently display a well-known reluctance to consult anyone about themselves, not wishing to be a nuisance, and their feet are often the first to deteriorate into a state of marked neglect. The need for chiropody must always be assessed because bunions and overgrown toenails will all contribute to instability and increase the risk of falling. Footwear should be inspected as it is often of the incorrect size or secondhand, with loose heels or worn soles. Attention should then be focused on the remainder of the patient's skin, and a careful examination made for ammoniacal rashes and then for pressure sores on the hips and heels which are easily missed.

The clinical detection of anaemia and metabolic disease is entirely unreliable in the elderly and so must always be supplemented with laboratory screening. Much information, however, can be obtained from the pulse and blood pressure and these are always of importance. Postural changes in the blood pressure should be looked for even when the resting blood pressure is high. Very often the apathetic patient, slumped in a chair with cold extremities, has an elevated blood pressure but with a marked postural drop. The descending colon and rectum must be assessed for faecal impaction and this will impart a characteristic odour to the faeces. A rectal examination is essential and it is best undertaken as a matter of routine. In men it permits the prostate to be felt and in women it may reveal a pelvic mass. A fairly simple examination is all that is necessary to find evidence of arthritis, hemiplegia or Parkinson's disease, and then attention must be directed to the patient's gait.

The examination of gait in an elderly patient is often much more informative than a conventional neurological examination, but it must always include asking the patient to rise from a chair and then to begin unstressed walking[35]. If this is normal the patient's individual degree of sway or unsteadiness can be measured on the ward by means of an ataxiameter. A broad-based unsteady gait with downgoing plantar responses, but with an absence of peripheral neuropathy or other neurological disease, is known as a frontal apraxia of gait. Active old people in hospital for conditions other than falls will make frequent errors in the placement of their feet which tend to disappear when the gait is speeded up[36]. On the other hand, elderly patients who have presented to hospital after a fall will invariably demonstrate increased errors with increased speed of walking.

Those gait abnormalities, which are the result of abnormal posture and deformities such as kyphosis and scoliosis, are generally easy to detect. Furthermore, there are several abnormalities of gait which are associated with much unsteadiness and these are usually the direct result of osteoarthritis. The shortening of a leg on account of an old femoral fracture or severe osteoarthrosis of the hip may cause a dipping gait. Unstable and peculiar gaits in which both legs are markedly externally rotated may be due to bilateral osteoarthrosis of the hips. Marked hip stiffness, again caused by advanced osteoarthrosis, may produce a gait which has been likened to walking a pair of protractors[37] – that is, small limited rocking movements. The lateral instability of a grossly disorganized knee, such as may be due to severe osteoarthritis, will sometimes result in an unsteady wobbling gait. Hobbling gaits are a consequence of painful feet and limping may be due to bone pain of various causes or intermittent claudication. Finally, gross unsteadiness with much lurching and staggering, but without the patient falling or otherwise sustaining injury, should always suggest a psychological disorder.

INVESTIGATIONS

Laboratory investigation will usually be required to complete the medical assessment of most elderly patients presenting with falls. It should initially take the form of a comprehensive screen for biochemical and haematological disorders which is then supplemented by specially chosen tests. It is important in the elderly that an estimation of thyroid function is included in the screening, because like anaemia the clinical impression of a thyroid disorder is often erroneous. Both hyperthyroidism and hypothyroidism are very satisfactory to treat and this may sometimes offer an old person a real chance to regain health. Further investigations are only indicated on an individual basis, but they should include an assessment for osteomalacia in every patient who presents with a fracture following a fall or a complaint of bone pain.

MANAGEMENT OF FRACTURES

Falls are virtually the exclusive cause of natural trauma in old age and overall about one in ten falls will result in a fracture (300 000 patients per year), and one in every 100 falls in the elderly will result in a fracture of the proximal femur (30 000 patients a year)[38]. A severe fracture in an elderly patient will invariably be associated with so many medical disorders that the surgery by itself will not be enough[39], no matter how well the technical procedures are undertaken. In isolation, the orthopaedic surgery will not be adequate to prevent an outcome of death in hospital, or permanently disabled old people and blocked orthopaedic beds as a direct consequence of these fractures. It has slowly become accepted that these problems can only be circumvented when the orthopaedic surgery is supplemented by the principles of geriatric medicine[40]. The essential features of a united approach to orthopaedic problems in the elderly are well illustrated by the management of fractures of the proximal femur because the treatment of these fractures is the key[41] to the management of all the other fractures that may occur in old age.

The most important tenet of geriatric orthopaedics is that elderly patients will be better served by walking than by immobility in bed, and as is the case for every kind of treatment for the elderly, those measures which do not promote mobility are generally discarded even where they happen to be the best methods of treatment for much younger patients[42]. After a fracture which has resulted in a serious loss of independence and in admission to hospital, rehabilitation including the repair of the fracture must be achieved without delay. If it is not, the elderly patient will not be given the best possible chance to regain his/her previous level of function and to return to his/her former life in the community.

In the example of a femoral fracture in an elderly person, it should follow that the fracture must always be repaired by means of an operation and that a technical method must be used which will allow the patient to bear weight as soon as recovery from the anaesthetic is complete. It is invariably feasible to repair a femoral fracture in the elderly, and those methods of operation which do not permit immediate postoperative weight-bearing are never employed because the need to immobilize the patient for several weeks in plaster must always be avoided.

Moreover, while a femoral fracture is unstable the nursing of an elderly patient will be extremely difficult because of immobility and incontinence, pain and confusion and the ever-present threat of pressure sores. It is therefore essential that femoral fractures in the elderly are secured by operation as early as possible, ideally no later than the first day after admission. On rare occasions a delay of not more than a few days is justified in order to mitigate the problems that are sometimes presented by cardiac failure or uncontrolled diabetes mellitus. A serious medical condition nevertheless is only a relative indication to postpone an operation for a short period, and it must never be accepted as a reason to refuse an operation, unless the patient is clearly about to die.

In essence the fundamental indications for the surgical repair of all fractures in old age are the presence of unremitting pain or a severe loss of personal independence as a direct result of the fracture. Elderly people withstand general anaesthesia and major orthopaedic operations remarkably well even when these are carried out as emergency procedures. Although old bones tend to break with ease because they lack mass, they also unite readily because the physiological function of the remaining bone is normal. Hence no old person should ever be excluded on the grounds of age alone from the relief of pain and the improvement in mobility which may be expected to follow an orthopaedic operation undertaken to repair an unstable fracture. Indeed patients with pathological fractures, and even those known to have an advanced degree of pre-existing dementia, should always have their fractured femurs secured by surgical repair, except when death seems inevitable within a day or two of falling down.

REHABILITATION AFTER FRACTURES

Whenever it is necessary to repair a fracture in an elderly patient a method of operation is chosen which will restore function to the injured part with the minimum of delay. In the example of fractures of the proximal femur a method of internal fixation is used that will allow all patients to sit out of bed for a short period on the first morning after operation and to start weight-bearing on the first postoperative day. Sometimes there may then be a temptation to advise that weight-bearing should be postponed after operation until bone healing with callous formation is seen on the radiographs, because the hold of an internal fixation is considered to be precarious. It is fundamental to the principles of geriatric orthopaedics that a delay in weight-bearing after operation must be resisted at all costs because it is entirely inappropriate in an elderly patient. It is far better to encourage these patients to mobilize normally, and then to repeat the operation if the fixation gives way, rather than to temporize and achieve bony union and risk rendering the patient helpless in the process.

Although this approach to rehabilitation is pragmatic, in practice it will seldom lead to further surgery perhaps because elderly people tend to stress a poor fixation far less than would be the case in younger patients. Nevertheless some difficulty in walking is almost universal after operation. This is only to be expected and most patients will in fact mobilize well during the first postoperative week. A serious lack of progress on the other hand will usually be due to pain and stiffness, severe loss of balance or generalized weakness[43].

Pain is seldom a problem in the immediate postoperative period, but some centres as a matter of routine provide epidural anaesthesia until the end of the second postoperative day. Severe and persistent pain, however, will produce a marked reluctance to weight-bear, and this must always be brought to the notice of the surgeon without delay because it may indicate a problem with the surgery.

After an operation almost all elderly patients will have stiffness which is relieved by early mobilization but when stiffness causes a failure to mobilize the presence of a stroke, Parkinsonism or arthritis is usually implied. In general, failure of a patient to walk after the repair of a femoral fracture is most commonly due to a serious impairment of balance. This is usually a part of the reason for the fall which led to the fracture, but it is not unknown for a cervical myelopathy to be caused by an inappropriate method of handling of the neck of the femur after the induction of anaesthesia. It is remarkable how many patients do manage nevertheless to regain adequate mobility during a short period of treatment with a low walking frame.

However, a failure to walk after an orthopaedic operation on account of generalized weakness is by far the more serious. It will invariably be the result of undetected illness which again will usually have preceded and led to the fall. It is vital that these patients are identified as early as possible in the first postoperative week and are then brought to the attention of a physician. If this stage in the patient's management is handled badly a long stay in hospital is inevitable. On the other hand if it is handled well the patient will often be able to return to the community.

Finally, although attention must inevitably focus on the injured part, and indeed it must be treated well, it is still the patient as a whole who ultimately matters. Therefore, the active involvement of every member of the rehabilitation team is of the utmost importance if an elderly patient recovering from a femoral fracture is to be given the best chance to achieve an early discharge home.

THE GERIATRIC ORTHOPAEDIC UNIT

Well-planned rehabilitation should enable over a half of elderly patients who have suffered a femoral fracture to leave hospital in less than a week. Most of these patients are active old people in whom the fracture was entirely the result of an accidental fall. They will sometimes require a period of further convalescence before they return to their homes. A few patients are already very frail individuals but they will be able nevertheless to return direct to a form of residental care. It is the remainder of elderly patients who threaten the efficient turnover in the orthopaedic wards, and if these patients are not managed well they will ultimately require a geriatric bed for long-stay care. They are patients in the main in whom the fall that led to the fracture was an expression of serious underlying illness, but some are patients for whom the postoperative recovery is not straight-forward. The sooner these patients are attended by a physician trained in geriatric medicine the better the outcome will be[44]. Moreover, there are many advantages to all concerned if these ill patients are separated out from the mainstream of the orthopaedic wards so that the rehabilitation and the treatment of their medical disorders can proceed in an appropriate environment[45].

For these reasons a system of joint care between the orthopaedic and geriatric services has been practised in Hastings for over 20 years in the form of the geriatric orthopaedic unit. There are other methods of the same collaboration and these may be equally as good but a combined unit will eventually represent a saving of beds both of the specialties involved.

Hastings is the centre of a retirement area where the proportion of people over 65 years of age in the population is more than twice the national average and where indeed 85 years is the mean age for patients with femoral fractures. Over 20 years ago a surgical ward which had been closed for lack of staff was reopened and at first ten beds were allocated to geriatric orthopaedics. Since that time the ward has been called the geriatric orthopaedic unit, and the principles on which the ward is run have not needed to change since they were originally defined[46].

The ward is situated in the same block as the ordinary acute geriatric wards and it is fundamental that the geriatricians undertake to provide the day-to-day care of the patients transferred to the unit from the orthopaedic wards. A patient on an orthopaedic ward is selected for transfer to the unit entirely at the discretion of the surgeon or the orthopaedic ward sister and they do not first have to ask the physician to take in the patient. Those patients who will be selected for transfer to the unit need to be identified as early as possible, and ideally they should be transferred during the first postoperative week. Sometimes the move to the unit is delayed because a bed is not available, and it is then most important that the patients waiting for transfer are assessed on the orthopaedic ward by the physician as early as possible. The move to the unit is always part of a carefully reasoned programme of rehabilitation and it is never undertaken for expediency alone. In general, the patients selected are those who are slow to get moving after operation, but the best criterion for selection is the degree of nursing care they require and this will usually reflect the presence of disease.

It is important to emphasize that the geriatric orthopaedic unit is for treatment alone and not for convalescence, but the majority of patients selected for transfer will invariably have problems exactly like those of elderly patients without fractures who are admitted to hospital as an emergency. Indeed, on arrival at the unit every patient is fully re-examined by the physicians and approached exactly as if he or she were newly admitted as emergencies to hospital.

The patients selected for transfer to the unit will remain under the clinical care of the orthopaedic surgeon and the physician in geriatric medicine for the entire duration of their stay in the ward. Apart from the separate ward rounds of the physician and the surgeon it is most important that the consultants of both departments see the patients together on a combined round undertaken at least once a week. The combined round is attended also by the junior medical staff from each department and by all the other members of the rehabilitation team. This arrangement is necessary to coordinate both the geriatric and the orthopaedic manage-ment in the individual patient and it will ensure that the patient receives the fullest consideration from both a remedial and social point of view. When a patient on the unit has outstayed the orthopaedic aspects of the treatment it is understood that he or she will be moved to an ordinary geriatric ward should this be requested by the orthopaedic surgeon. In practice this is seldom required because the majority of patients are able to return direct to the community after spending about 3 weeks in the unit, and overall less than 5% of patients eventually require long-stay care in the geriatric wards. This system of orthopaedic geriatric partnership has a worked well for over 20 years, and has led to a better outcome for the patients and a better use of hospital resources by the staff.

Acknowledgements

This chapter is the work of a multidisciplinary team. While our librarian Mrs Anne Taylor searched through the literature with remarkable skill and unearthed many hidden articles, another expert, Mrs E. Hodge sat typing for a long time and then coordinated the production of the manuscript. Any wisdom transmitted by the content is only a small part of that received from Dr R. E. Irvine and all the therapists in the Department of Medicine for the Elderly.

References

1. Fenton Lewis, A. (1981). Fractured neck of femur, the changing incidence. *Br. Med. J.*, **283**, 1217.
2. Duthie Report (1981). DHSS. Orthopaedic services: Report of a Working Party to The Secretary of State for Social Services. (London: HMSO).
3. Campbell, A. J. (1976). Femoral neck fractures in elderly women: a prospective study. *Age Ageing*, **5**, 102.
4. Naylor, M. B. and Rosin A. S. (1970). Falling as a cause of admission to a geriatric unit. *Practitioner*, **205**, 327–30.
5. Lucht, U. (1971). A prospective study of accidental falls and injuries in the home among elderly people. *Acta Socio-med. Scand.*, **3**, 105.

6. Sheldon, J. H. (1960). The natural history of falls in old age. *Br. Med. J.*, **2**, 1658–90.
7. Registrar General for England and Wales (1978). *Annual Report*. (London: HMSO).
8. Azar, G. J. and Lawton, A. H. (1964). Gait and stepping as factors in frequent falls of elderly women. *Gerontologia*, **4**, 83–4.
9. Gallannaugh, S. C., Martin, A. and Millard, P. H. (1976). Regional survey of fractured neck of femur. *Br. Med. J.*, **2**, 1496–7.
10. Mark, I. and Bebington, P. (1976). Space phobia syndrome or agoraphobic variant. *Br. Med. J.*, **2**, 345–7.
11. Howell, T. H. (1971). Old folk who fall. *Practitioner*, **175**, 56–8.
12. Knowelder, J., Buhr, A. J. and Dunbar, O. (1964). The incidence of fractures in people over 35 years of age. *Br. J. Soc. Prev. Med.*, **18**, 130.
13. Exton-Smith, A. N. (1976). For people in their sixties fracture and falls are a special hazard. *Modern Geriatr.*, Vol. 6, **7**, 27–30.
14. Evans, J. C., Prudham, D. and Wandless, I. (1979). A prospective study of fractured proximal femur. *Pub. Hlth.*, **93**, 235–41.
15. Wild, D., Isaacs, B. and Nayak, U. S. L. (1980). How dangerous are falls in old people at home? *Br. Med. J.*, **282**, 266–8.
16. Remakus, B. L. (1981). How to prevent confusion in the elderly. *Geriatrics*, **36**, 121–5.
17. Gryfe, C. I., Amies, A. and Ashley, M. I. (1977). A longitudinal study of falls in an elderly population, incidence and morbidity. *Age Ageing*, **6**, 201–10.
18. Devas, M. (1977). Introduction to fractures in the elderly. In Devas, M. E. (ed.) *Geriatric Orthopaedics*. (London: Academic Press).
19. Strouthidis, T. M. and Irvine, R. E. (1977). Medical care in geriatric orthopaedics. In Devas, M. E. (ed.) *Geriatric Orthopaedics*, pp. 9, 20. (London: Academic Press).
20. Wild, D., Isaacs, B. and Nayak, U. S. L. (1980). It is estimated that three million fall each year. How dangerous are falls in old people at home? *Br. Med. J.*, **282**, 266–8.
21. Wilson Barnett, J. (1979). *Stress in Hospital*. (London: Churchill Livingstone).
22. Davies, A. D. (1983). Stresses of hospitalisation in the elderly: nurses and patients perceptions. *J. Adv. Nurs.*, **8**, 99–105.
23. Fernsebner, B. (1983). Sleep deprivation in patients. *Aorn.*, J., **37**, 35–42.
24. Nabarro, J. (1984). Unrecognised psychiatric illness in medical patients. *Br. Med. J.*, **289**, 635–6.
25. Couchman, M. E. (1975). Unpublished management report. Nursing Office, St Helen's Hospital, Hastings.
26. Wilcox, G. K. and Middleton, A. M. (1980). *Geriatrics*. (London: Grant McIntyre).
27. Brocklehurst, J. C., Exton-Smith, A. N., Lempert-Barber, S. M., Hunt, L. P. and Palmer, M. K. (1978). Fracture of femur in old age. *Age Ageing*, **7**, 7–15.
28. Isaacs, B, (1983). Falls in old age. In Hinchcliffe, R. (ed.) *Hearing Disorders in the Elderly*. (London: Churchill Livingstone).
29. Isaacs, B. (1980). Guidelines for reducing the risk of disability. *Geriatr. Med.*, **Feb.**
30. Wild, D., Isaacs, B. and Nayak, U. S. L. (1980). How dangerous are falls in old people at home? *Br. Med. J.*, **282**, 266–88.
31. Droller, H. and Pemberton, J. (1953). Vertigo in a random sample of elderly people living at home. *J. Laryngol. Otol.*, **67**, 689–94.
32. Hinchcliffe, R. (1983). Epidemiology of balance disorders in the elderly. In *Hearing and Balance in the Elderly*. (London: Churchill Livingstone).
33. Strouthidis, T. M. and Irvine, R. E. (1977). Medical Care in Geriatric Orthopaedics. p. 20. (London: Academic Press).
34. Garland, M. (1978). Falls. *Hosp. Update*, **4**, 4.
35. Adams, G. (1978). *Essentials of Geriatric Medicine*. (Oxford: Oxford Medical Publications).
36. Guimaraes, R. M. and Isaacs, B. (1980). Characteristics of gait in old people who fall. *Int. Rehab. Med.*, **2**, 177–80.
37. Hodkinson, H. M. (1980). *Common Symptoms of Disease in the Elderly*. (Oxford: Blackwell Scientific Publications).
38. Evans, J. G. (1979). Fractured proximal femur in Newcastle upon Tyne. *Age Ageing*, **8**, 16–24.
39. Clark, A. N. G. and Wainwright, D. (1966). The management of fractured neck of

femur in the elderly female: a joint approach of orthopaedic surgery and geriatric medicine. *Geront. Clin.*, **8,** 321.

40. Irvine, R. E. and Devas, M. E. (1964). *Fractured Neck of Femur in Elderly Women
    Age with a Future.* (Copenhagen: Munksgaard).
41. Devas, M. B. (1964). Fractures in the elderly. *Geront. Clin.*, **6,** 347–59.
42. Devas, M. B. (1974). Geriatric orthopaedics. *Br. Med. J.*, **1,** 190–2.
43. Wright, W. E. and Fenwick, G. M. (1978). The fractured femur: why call in the geriatri-
    cian? *Injury*, **9,** 282.
44. Irvine, R. E. and Devas, M. B. (1969). The geriatric orthopaedic unit. *Br. J. Geriatr.
    Pract.*, **6,** 19–25.
45. Irvine, R. E. and Strouthidis, T. M. (1977). The geriatric orthopaedic unit. In Devas,
    M. B. (ed.) *Geriatric Orthopaedics.* (London: Academic Press).
46. Devas, M. B. and Irvine, R. E. (1963). The geriatric orthopaedic unit. *J. Bone Jt. Surg.*,
    46B, 630.

Index

133